IMAGES
of America

NORWICH STATE HOSPITAL

On the Cover: This 1931 photograph of Norwich State Hospital looks toward the southern end of the campus, with the Administration Building in front and Ward A South, later known as Salmon, in the rear. The ornate original portico on the Administration Building was removed around 1960. (Courtesy of Preston Historical Society.)

IMAGES
of America

NORWICH STATE HOSPITAL

Christine M. Rockledge
Introduction by Steve DePolito

ARCADIA
PUBLISHING

ISBN 978-1-4671-2962-6

Published by Arcadia Publishing
Charleston, South Carolina

Library of Congress Control Number: 2018939495

For all general information, please contact Arcadia Publishing:
Telephone 843-853-2070
Fax 843-853-0044
E-mail sales@arcadiapublishing.com
For customer service and orders:
Toll-Free 1-888-313-2665

Visit us on the Internet at www.arcadiapublishing.com

This book is dedicated to all the former employees and patients of Norwich State Hospital. You leave behind a proud legacy that will never be forgotten.

Contents

Acknowledgments 6

Introduction 7

1. From Near Failed Beginnings 9
2. Institutional Ups and Downs 33
3. Hospital Changes and World War II 59
4. Norwich State Hospital on the International Map 73
5. The People of Norwich State Hospital 99

ACKNOWLEDGMENTS

The near decade spent delving into Norwich State Hospital's past has blessed me with meeting countless generous and beautiful people. Without Lloyd Langhammer, Carol Burns McDermott, Patti Daniels, Patty Nichols and Steven Falade, Heather Angel, Jacki John, and everyone in the Norwich Hospital (NH) family, the missing pieces I had been searching for to complete the puzzle that this lengthy project became could never have been found. My gratitude to you and everyone in the Norwich Hospital family is infinite. Every individual I have met along this journey has so generously reopened their lives at Norwich State Hospital through their memories and personal photographs so I could portray what their beloved institution was like as accurately as possible.

Enormous thanks go to Steve DePolito for coming back to Norwich State Hospital (NSH) one last time. Your dedication and support to this project has been invaluable. This book could not have been completed without an NSH employee's touch.

Special thanks are extended to Linda Christensen of the Preston Historical Society for her generosity and support. Personal thanks are extended to Kevin Thibdeau and Alexis Guermeur for keeping the fire alive, Brian Dias for putting up with me, Dave Walsh and Cathy for memories I treasure dearly, and especially Kristen Polci-Parsons for always believing in me and always being there for me. Kristen, I will never break my promise.

Over 20 years have passed since the closure of Norwich State Hospital. Gradually, the buildings are diminishing and employees don't work together anymore, but their closeness still remains as though NSH were still open. As an outsider looking in, all the years I spent sitting among former employees and listening to their stories and watching them laugh and reminisce together, it is evident that the family formed all those years ago is as alive today as the history and memory of Norwich State Hospital always will be. This book would not exist without you.

May the future developers of the Norwich State Hospital property preserve, honor, and do justice to one of Connecticut's most caring and venerable landmarks and to the generations of families that were formed on those grounds over nearly 100 years.

INTRODUCTION

When the Norwich State Hospital closed its doors on October 10, 1996, I was there. As clinical coordinator of the substance abuse services, I was tasked with supervising the closing of the Gallup Building. It was a sad day for patients and staff alike. For many patients, Norwich State Hospital was considered a home—a safe place to be. For staff, the employees and patients at Norwich State Hospital were like a big family

In 2004, I began work on a public access television project on Norwich State Hospital. The result was an hour-long video documentary titled *Brewster's Neck: Memories of Norwich State Hospital.* It was completed in time for the 10th anniversary of the hospital's closing and received favorable reviews from the local media. This video project was produced with the intent of showing that good was done at the hospital, while acknowledging that abuses that occurred within all mental institutions across the country did also happen at Norwich. Three years later, I edited VHS tape recordings made by NSH police to produce the video *Last Day at Norwich State Hospital.* This video project gave viewers the opportunity to see portions of the tunnels and inside some of the buildings, and what the exterior of the vast campus looked like on the day we said goodbye. While I was generally pleased with both projects, I was frustrated with the fact that I could not objectively present a historical documentary on the hospital. After all, I was still working in the field and too close to the topic. I was also getting increasingly annoyed with the public misconceptions of what NSH was all about. It seemed like all people wanted to hear were horror stories of haunted asylums and horrific abuses. I was tired and frustrated at work. My last two years as a clinical social worker involved working with the homeless and mentally ill, many of whom used to call NSH home. I resigned myself to the fact that I had probably had gone as far as I could go in presenting the story of Norwich State Hospital. When I retired in 2014 from the State of Connecticut, I tried to put it all in the past. Then, Christine Rockledge contacted me to say she was doing a second Norwich State Hospital book.

I first met Christine in 2011. At that time, she was doing research on Norwich State Hospital for her first book, the independently published *More Patience, Less Patients*, and came across a copy of *Brewster's Neck* at the Otis Library in Norwich. The library staff contacted me for her, and I agreed to be interviewed. While her first book was locally successful, she obviously felt a need to say more. Consequently, she has authored this book, a complete history of the Norwich State Hospital. This is the book I hoped and prayed would be written. A carefully researched, objective look at the history of the hospital, the patients who lived there, and the staff who worked there. As soon as I started reading chapter one, I was immediately reminded of the little bit of history I heard about years ago from former superintendent Garrell Mullaney regarding the Maine Insane Hospital. In 1840, the Maine Insane Hospital was opened in Augusta, Maine, one of the first of its kind in the United States. The hospital was built across the river from the capitol building. The reason for this was so that the governor and the legislature would never forget the hospital. I remember thinking that she nailed it—right on the first page! The whole concept of a "state hospital" is dependent on what the state deems necessary and appropriate, based on political agendas and financial resources. And the care of the mentally ill has never been at the top of any legislative agenda.

In this book, you will read much about the Norwich Hospital family; family, of course, usually refers to parents, children, siblings, and spouses, but can also mean, as defined by Merriam-Webster, "a group of people united by certain convictions or a common affiliation." At Norwich Hospital, it was the culture of caring that was passed through generations that defined the Norwich Hospital family. For me, like many others who worked there, I was part of a second generation of hospital workers. My mom was a nurse. Dad worked in food service. Uncle Tom worked in the storeroom. Uncle Ed and Aunt Katherine worked in laundry. Aunt Ellen, my mom's sister, was a social worker in charge of the adolescent unit. I remember going to visit Mom's patients in the Lippitt Building, which was the medical unit at the time. It was Halloween 1964; I was five years old, all dressed up in costume. As a kid, I remember walking through the main kitchen with Dad on many occasions. I remember Mom bringing us kids to the hospital's reservoir beach. It was the 1960s, and I had no idea that someday I would be working with many of the other kids on the beach. When Mom passed away in 1972 at the age of 36, the hospital family gave Dad much-needed support. Seven years later, Dad married my stepmom Barbara, who worked in food service and whose own mother was a psychiatric aide. In 1981, I began my own career at the hospital as a psychiatric aide. Three years later, after a stint in the Army, my brother Gary also became a psych aide. Like my dad, I married a nurse I met when we worked the detox unit in 1986; Sherri and I have been together since. By the time Norwich Hospital closed, I had 38 years of photographs along with memories burned into my brain.

When I reviewed Christine's book for the first time, I was amazed by how she brought the past back to life with carefully researched narrative and pictures. Many of these pictures have never been published—some of them I am seeing for the first time. She illustrates the legacy of caring and community while not shying away from the dark side of Norwich State Hospital's history. This book is important in that it will provide future generations with an accurate, complete picture of what the Norwich State Hospital was all about, from inception to closing. I am honored to have been asked to write this introduction and am confident that this book will portray the true spirit of Norwich State Hospital.

—Steven DePolito, MS, MSW
March 2018

One

From Near Failed Beginnings

Norwich State Hospital's origin dates to 1890. Connecticut had only one public institution at the time, Connecticut Hospital for the Insane, to care for the state's population of mentally ill. Its patient census was in excess of its capacity, and its staff found it impossible to accommodate new admissions while safely and comfortably housing the existing population. Concerned with present and projected overcrowding problems, a special investigative committee was designated by the General Assembly. Its task was to find a solution to the problem by either building expansion at the Connecticut Hospital for the Insane or the establishment of a new institution elsewhere in the state. The committee determined that for the patients' benefit and for long-term economic feasibility, a new state hospital elsewhere should be established.

The Connecticut legislature did not act upon the committee's recommendation. Connecticut Hospital for the Insane's census continued to climb and conditions became more claustrophobic on the wards. The hospital reiterated its concerns about the state's present and future increase of the "insane" population in 1895. The request for either new ward buildings or the establishment of a new state hospital was repeated. The request was denied. The legislature instead authorized renovating existing buildings on the campus to rectify the problem.

This solution proved unsatisfactory, and again, the hospital was filled beyond its capacity.

The matter landed before the legislature for a third time in 1897. The city of Norwich offered to donate a tract of land for the new state hospital. Considering this donation, the General Assembly appointed a special committee to investigate the desirability of the site. Its findings were reported to the legislature of 1899. While the representatives unanimously agreed that additional accommodations for the state's mentally ill were desperately needed, they were not unanimous in agreeing that a second institution be established. The bill was defeated.

It was resubmitted again in 1901 only to meet with a like fate.

Two more years passed before the General Assembly agreed that a second state institution was necessary and "An Act Establishing a State Hospital for the Insane at Norwich" was approved on June 12, 1903.

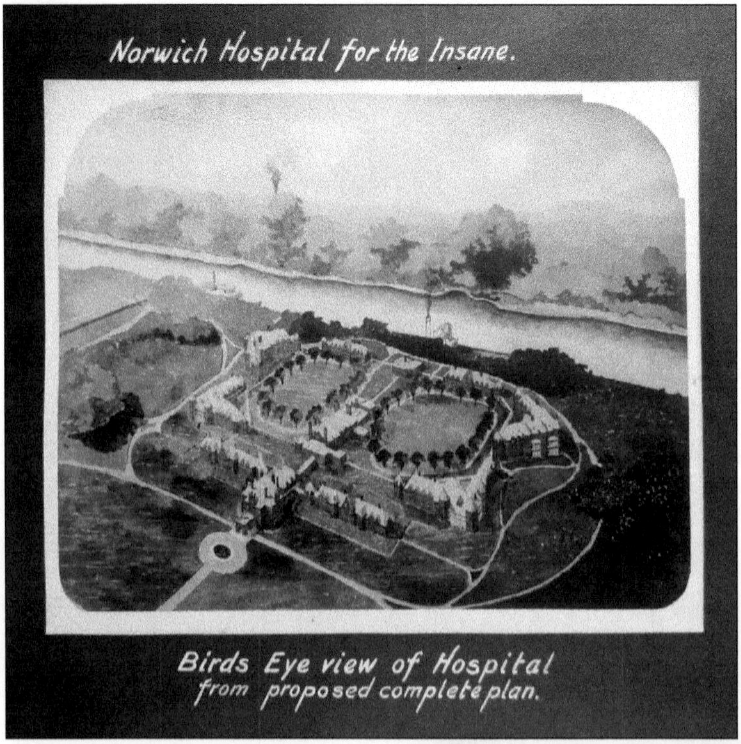
Norwich Hospital for the Insane.
Birds Eye view of Hospital
from proposed complete plan.

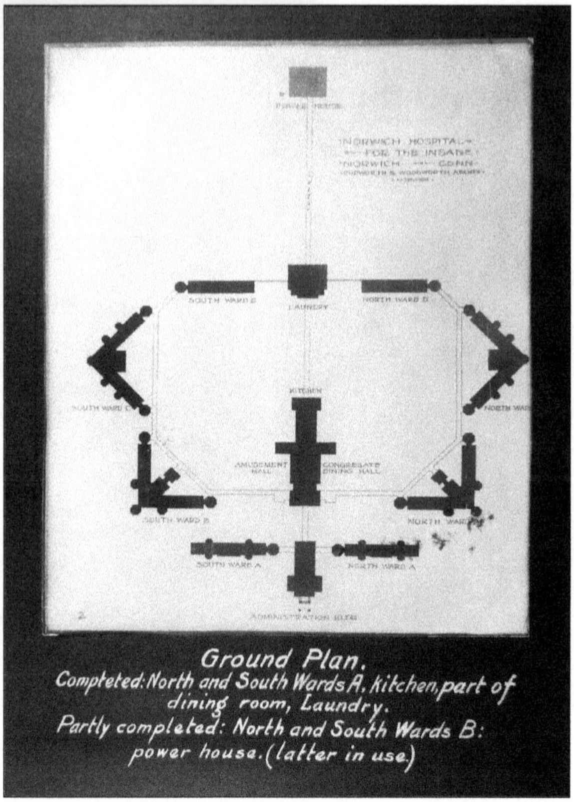

Upon the passing of the act to establish the Norwich Hospital for the Insane, Norwich architectural firm Cudworth & Woodworth was selected to design the new state hospital. Cudworth & Woodworth were responsible for many of Norwich's most impressive buildings, such as the Chelsea Savings Bank Building, two buildings on the Norwich Free Academy campus, and numerous others in and around the city. Proposals and plans for the new hospital were rapidly drawn. The c. 1903 artist's conception of the campus, pictured above, shows a bird's-eye view of the proposed completed hospital. The image at right illustrates the manner in which the campus was to be neatly and efficiently laid out. Construction of the Norwich Hospital for the Insane began on October 28, 1903. (Both, courtesy of Connecticut State Library.)

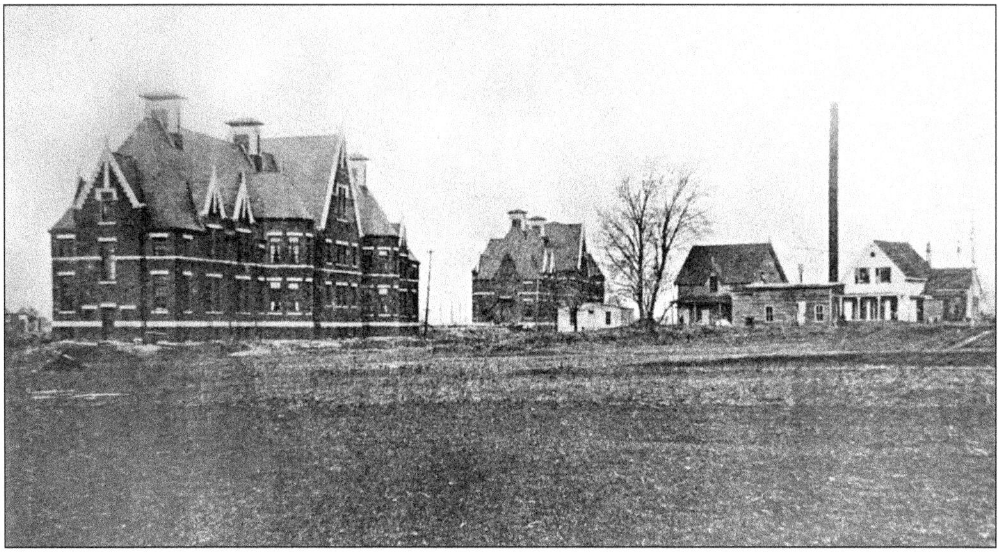

The work was carried out with the utmost perseverance. On October 10, 1904, the Norwich Hospital for the Insane opened with the admittance of its first patient. Upon opening, however, the first two ward buildings, Wards A North and South, pictured above, were not immediately ready for occupancy. The accompanying farmhouses also shown above were acquired with the property and served as a temporary laundry and kitchen. A temporary powerhouse was erected between them. The first patient was admitted to the superintendent's home, a short distance from the main hospital site, until the ward buildings were furnished later that month. The superintendent's home also served as a temporary administration building. The hospital was formally opened with official ceremonies in December of that year. The photograph below shows Ward A North, completed and occupied a few months later in 1904. (Above, courtesy of Connecticut State Library; below, courtesy of Preston Historical Society.)

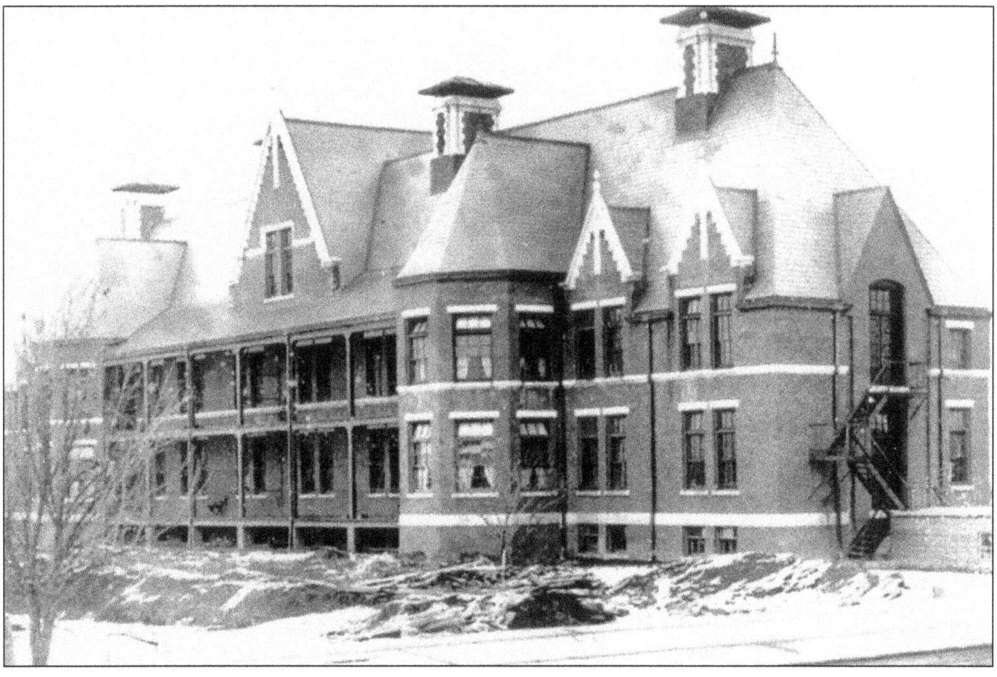

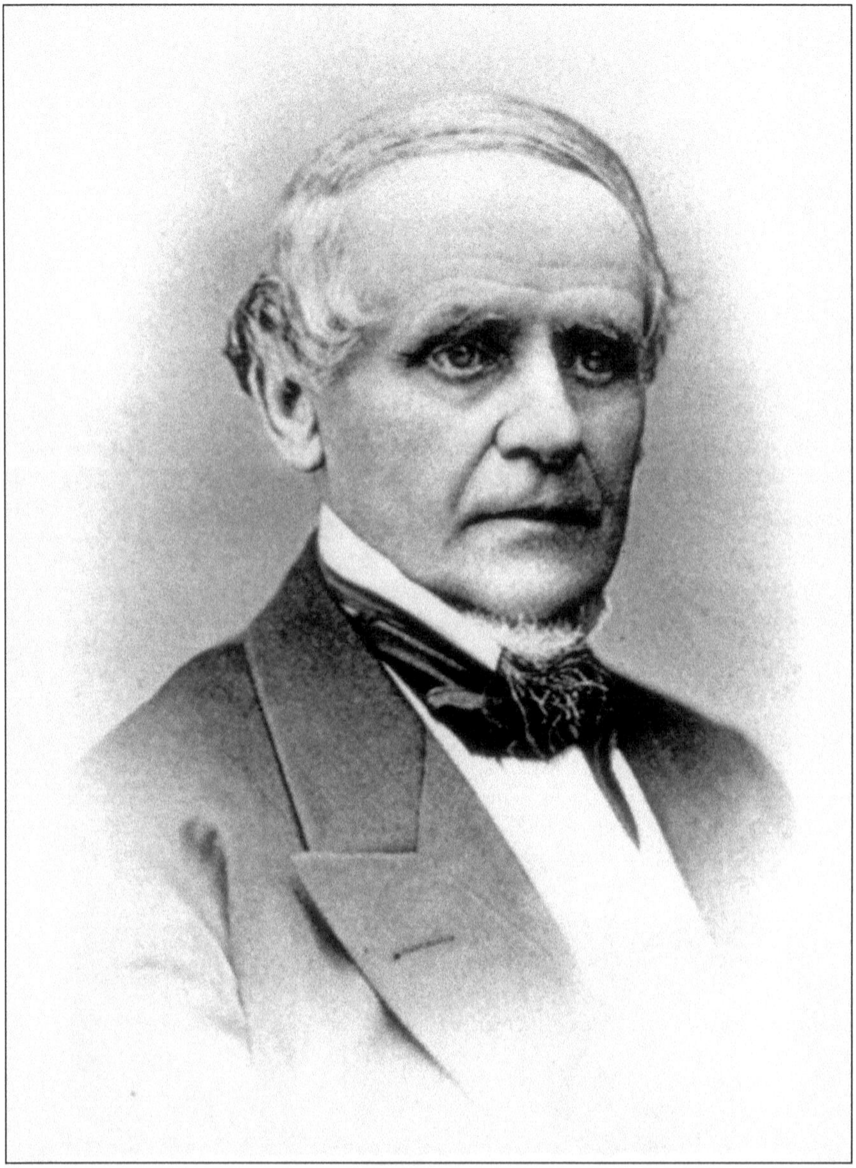

To understand Norwich State Hospital and its unique building arrangement, one must understand the standards and trends of asylum construction during the late 19th and early 20th centuries. Prior to the end of the 19th century, large, sprawling castle-like single-structure buildings known as Kirkbride buildings were the favored standard for asylum construction. These tremendous structures grew from a concept in therapeutic architectural design conceived by Dr. Thomas Story Kirkbride. Dr. Kirkbride, seen here, was an advocate for moral treatment therapy and believed the designs of his buildings, which boasted scenic views of lavish grounds and plenty of sunlight and fresh air from all sides, was highly conducive to the treatment of and recovery from mental illness. Kirkbride buildings featured a central administration building flanked by two wings. Patients were classified and placed according to gender and illness. Male patients were housed in one wing, with female patients in the other. Each wing was subdivided into tiered wards. The quietest, most well-behaved patients were housed closest to the administrative section, while the noisier, more disturbed patients were in the wards at the rear of the building. (Author's collection.)

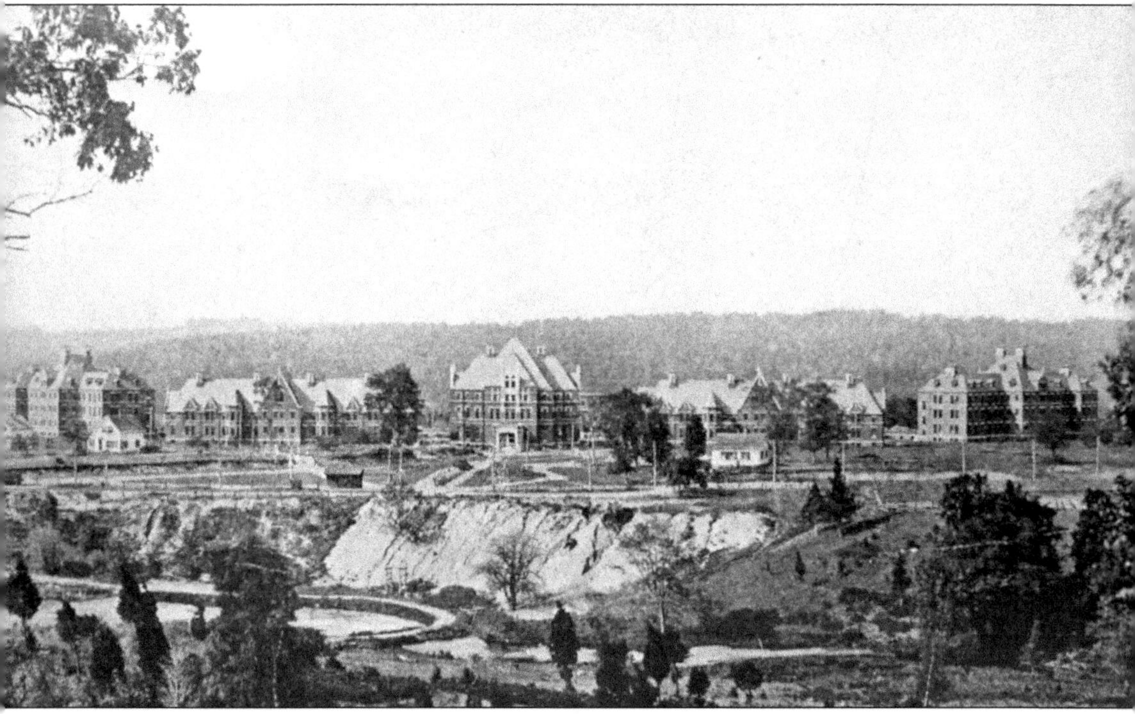

Psychiatric hospital structures from the late 19th century into the early 20th century were designed and constructed strategically to not create a frightful, menacing appearance. Asylums appeared lavish and were spread out over park-like grounds that boasted magnificent views and beautifully detailed buildings. The idea behind this was to create a visually pleasing atmosphere believed to be more conducive to treatment and recovery and to avoid giving the institution's patients, staff, and visitors the impression that they were in a place of punishment. Prior to the turn of the 20th century, Kirkbride buildings were being phased out in favor of smaller, separate buildings. Kirkbride's ideals were not completely abandoned in the planning and erection of the Norwich Hospital for the Insane. The hospital was an amalgam of both Kirkbride's ideas and the newer, more modern cottage-style construction. Norwich State Hospital, pictured in 1908, sat upon the eastern banks of the Thames River in East Norwich, now known as Preston, Connecticut. Its original 172 acres lie in an area known as Brewster's Neck, a name that would later become locally synonymous with the hospital. (Courtesy of Connecticut State Library.)

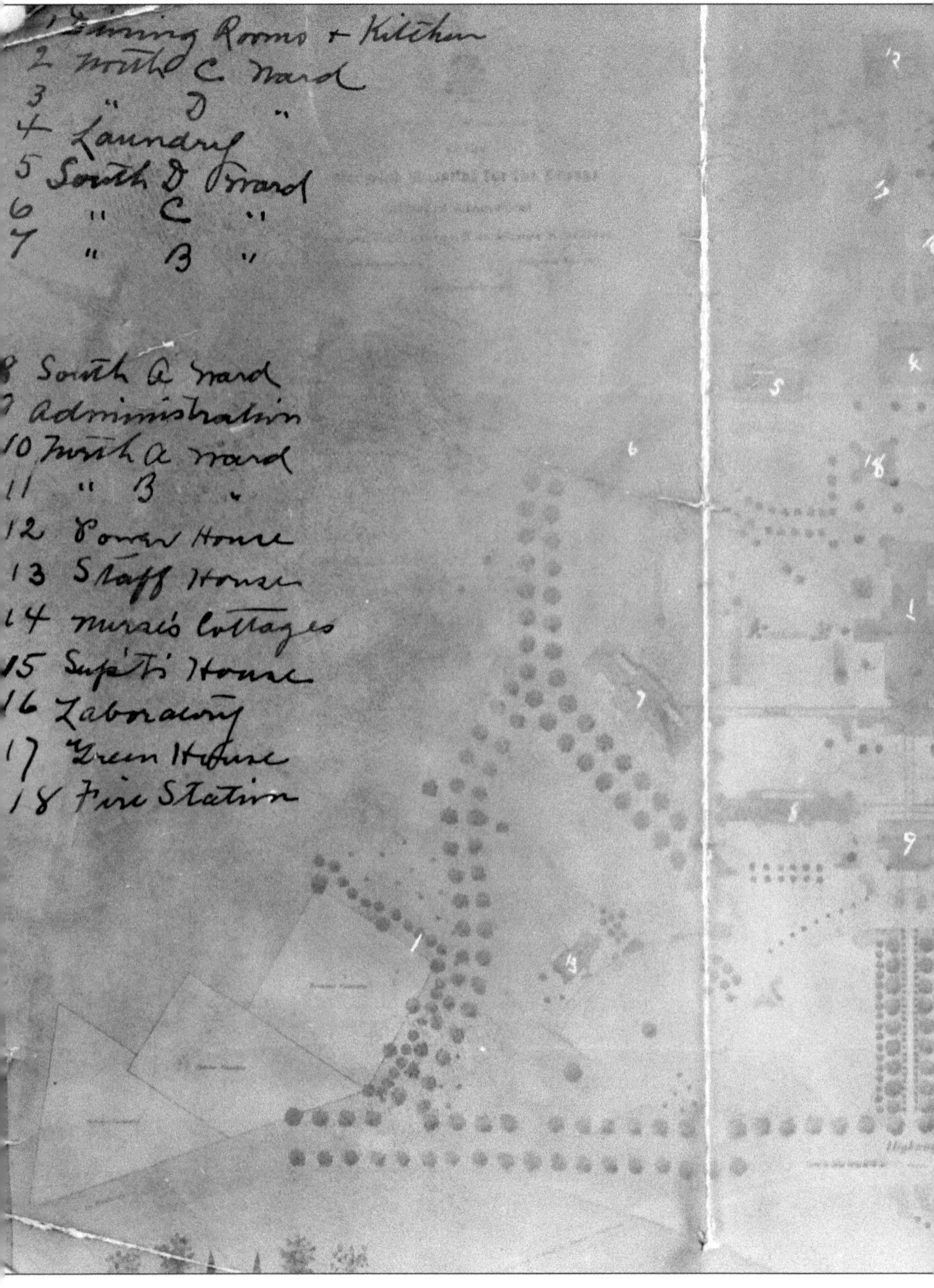
1 Dining Rooms + Kitchen
2 North C. Ward
3 " D "
4 Laundry
5 South D Ward
6 " C "
7 " B "
8 South A Ward
9 Administration
10 North A Ward
11 " B "
12 Power House
13 Staff House
14 Nurse's Cottages
15 Sup't's House
16 Laboratory
17 Green House
18 Fire Station

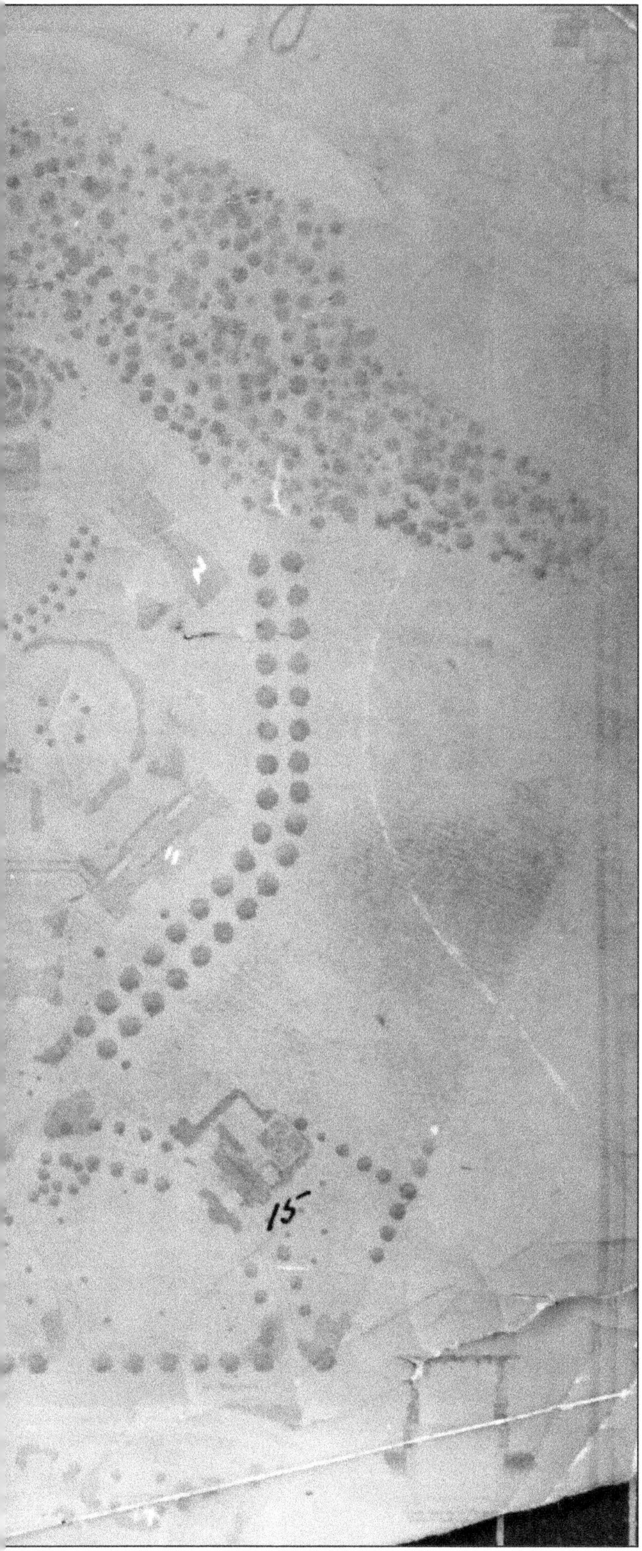

This early grounds map from 1912 depicts the completed building arrangement of the hospital. A French Gothic–style administration building sat slightly front and center as the hospital's first impression. The Administration Building was flanked by two wards of similar architectural style originally designed for well-behaved patients. Later ward buildings were of Colonial Revival style. Ward buildings for the more boisterous, difficult, and violent patients were at the rear of the campus. The hospital's ward buildings were arranged in the shape of a half-square extending from the front of the property to the rear on either side. In comparison to a Kirkbride building, these two sides were the "wings" of the hospital. Female and male patients were housed in pairs of identical buildings on either side, one denoted as the north wing and the other as the south wing. (Courtesy of Connecticut State Library.)

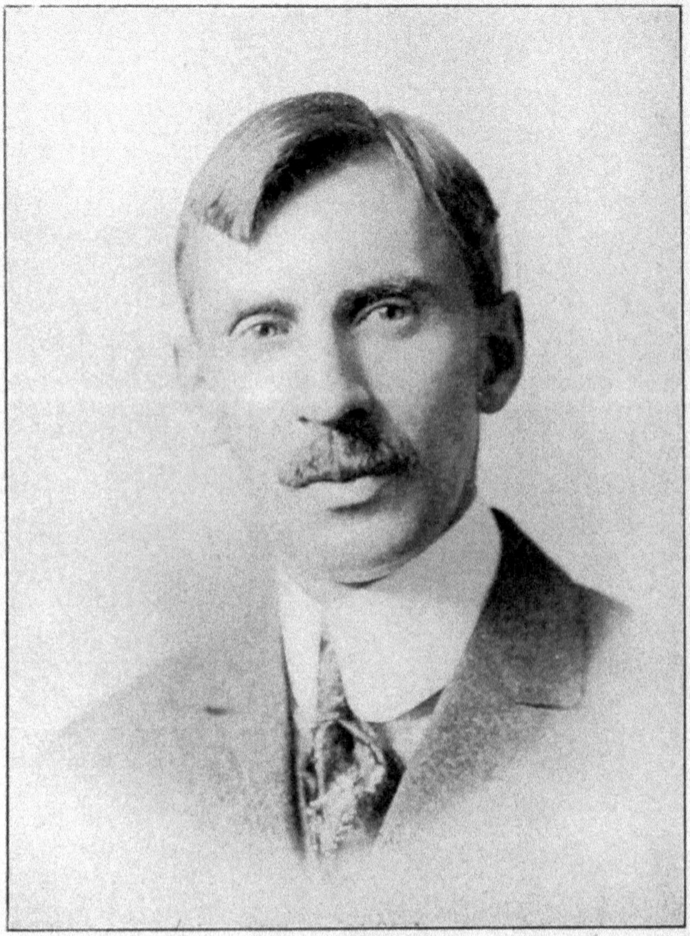

HENRY M. POLLOCK, M.D.

Dr. Henry M. Pollock, seen here, was the first active superintendent of Norwich Hospital for the Insane. His predecessor, Dr. Jonathan H. Allen, was chosen as the first superintendent but only held the office for six months. Dr. Pollock hailed from Fergus Falls State Hospital in Minnesota. He was a homeopathic physician with a great deal of respect, compassion, and dedication to the mentally ill. He detested the public's negative attitude that treated mentally ill persons as though they were criminals. From the beginning of his tenure, he resented the word "insane" being attached to the hospital's name and repeatedly advocated before the General Assembly for the name to be changed to Norwich State Hospital. Dr. Pollock commanded the state's respect for the mentally ill knowing this would filter down to the community. During his second appeal for the name to be changed, he stated, "Prisons are becoming known as reformatories and correctional institutions as schools. The insane, as a class, are sensitive, and their relatives particularly so." His requests were continuously denied. (Author's collection.)

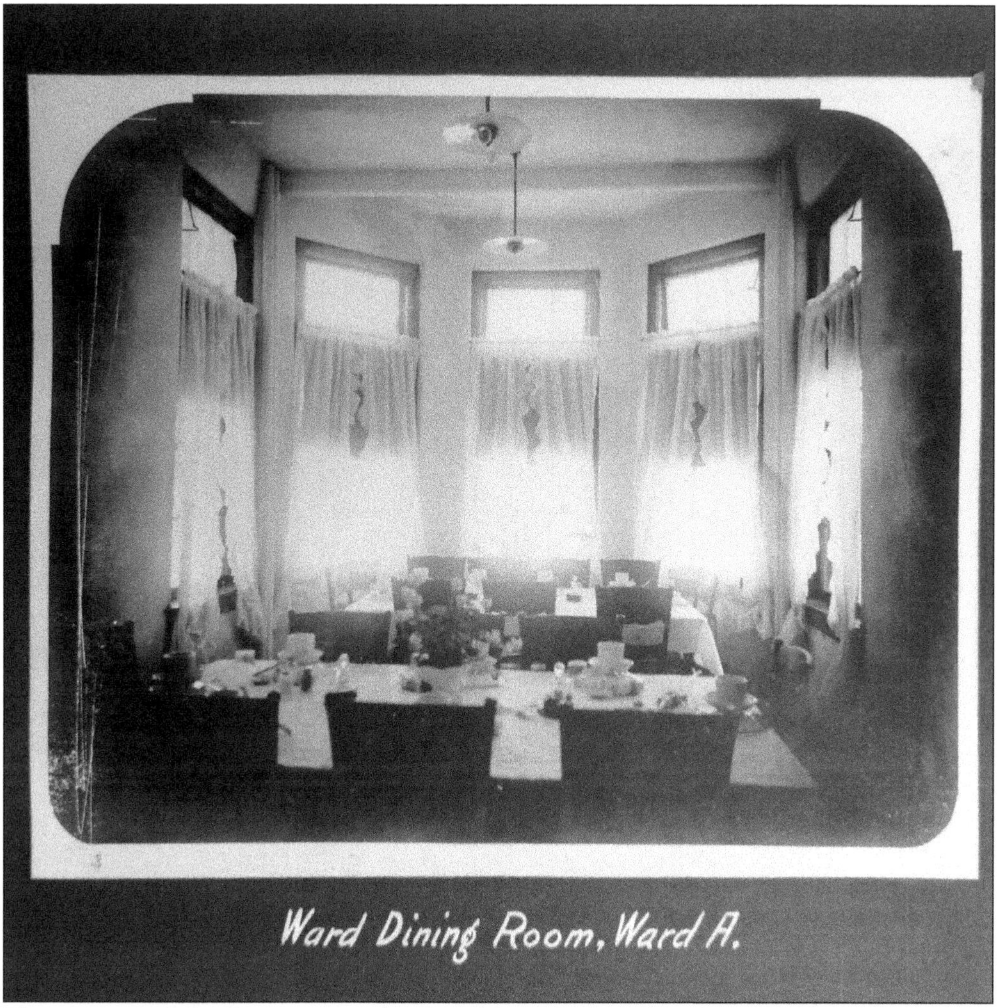

The interiors of the first two completed and furnished ward buildings, Wards A North and South, were adorned with detailed and delicate home-style furnishings. According to both Dr. Kirkbride and Dr. Pollock's beliefs, creating a homelike surrounding was highly advantageous to patients' comfort, happiness, and chance of recovery. Wards A North and South were designed to house 50 patients each. Between transfers from the Connecticut Hospital for the Insane and local admissions, Norwich Hospital for the Insane was overcrowded in excess of 70 patients by the end of the hospital's first biennial period of 1906. (Courtesy of Connecticut State Library.)

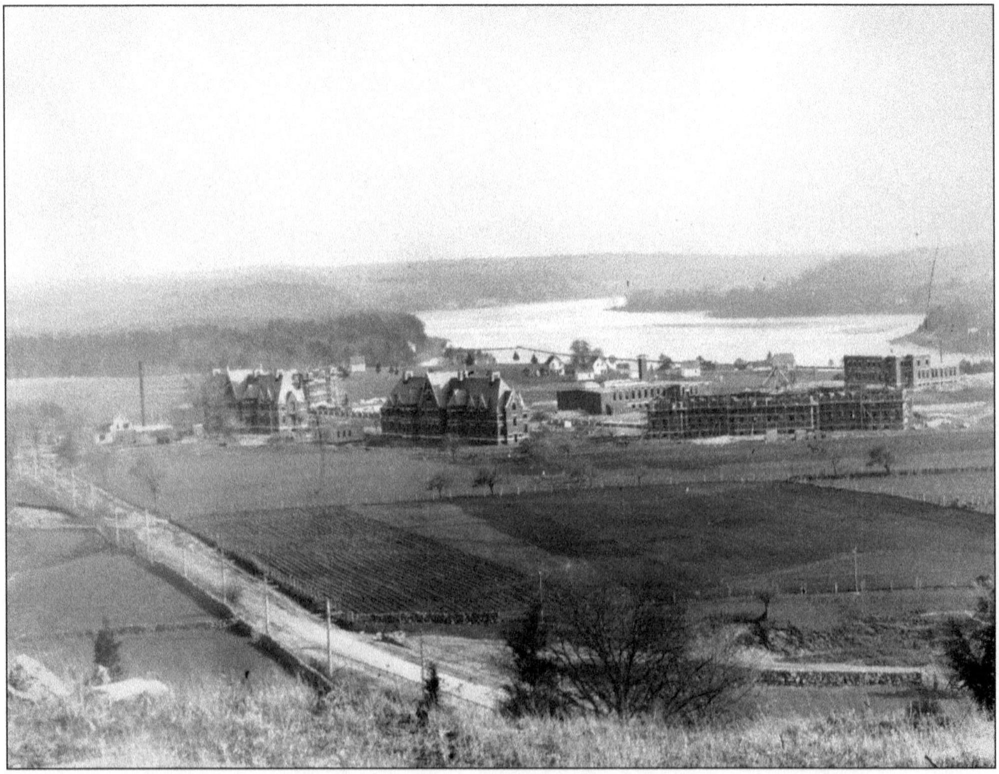

At the end of 1906, the next wards awaiting completion, Wards B North and South, were behind schedule due to opposition from the General Assembly in appropriating adequate funds to complete them. The Norwich Hospital for the Insane Board of Trustees stressed to the governor that due to the immediate overcrowding the hospital faced upon opening, new admissions could only be received as vacancies occurred until these two new ward buildings were complete. The photograph below was taken the same day as the one above and shows the completed Wards A from the rear and the construction of Ward B South in 1906. When completed, these wards were each three stories in height and built to accommodate 300 patients. (Above, author's collection; below, courtesy of Preston Historical Society.)

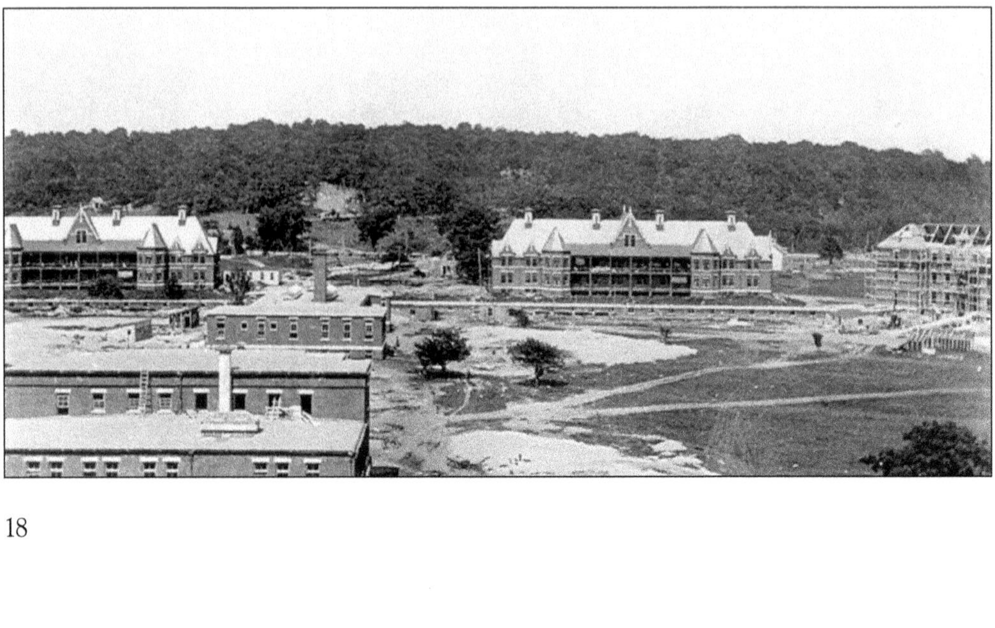

This temporary office building was erected around 1906 adjacent to Ward A North. The building contained a reception room for receiving patients, administrative offices, and a pharmacy. A proper administration building would later sit next to this temporary building. Before the temporary structure was built, Dr. Pollock received patients in two rooms of his cottage on the hospital grounds. (Author's collection.)

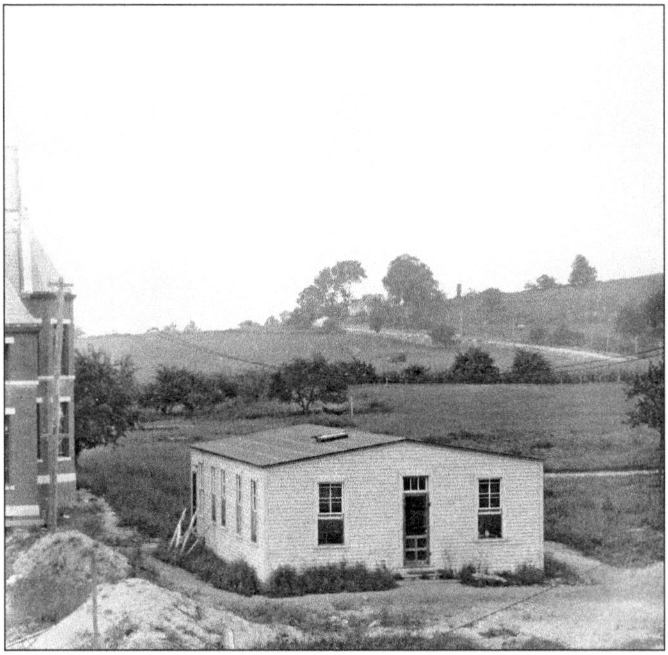

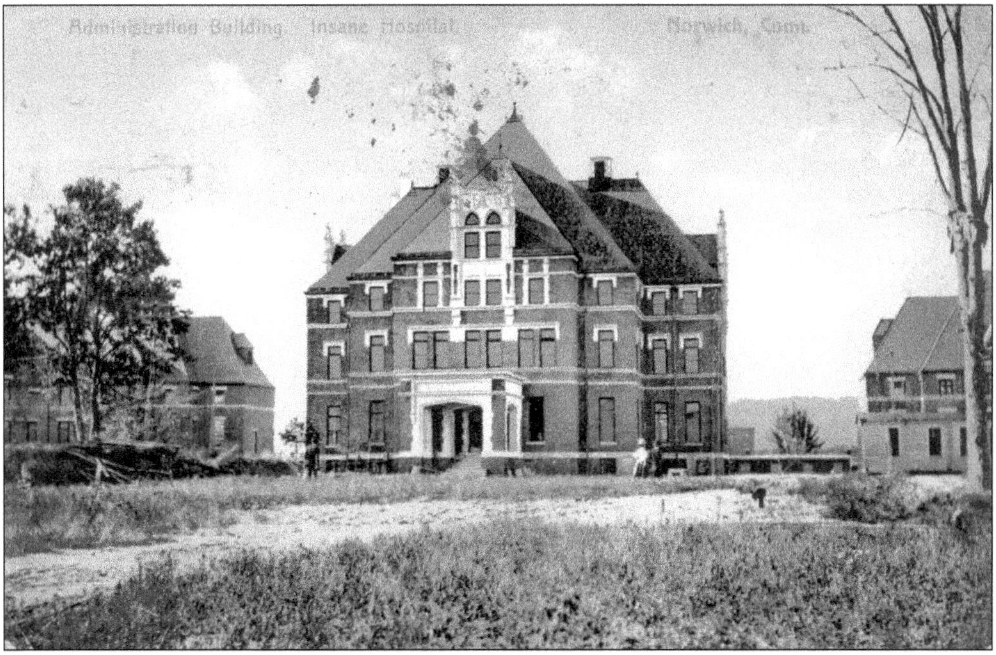

The Administration Building, shown in this 1910 postcard, was completed in 1908. The first floor contained a reception hall, reception room, patient library, pharmacy, and offices for the superintendent, staff, business, and clinical assistants. The second floor housed the trustees' room, committee room, staff library, photographic room with adjoining darkroom, and operating suites comprised of anesthetic, surgeon's dressing, and sterilizing rooms. The third floor was occupied by separate psychopathic wards, known as "Center Hospital," for the reception and treatment of patients. Until the amusement hall was completed in 1912, a makeshift amusement hall also occupied the third floor. (Author's collection.)

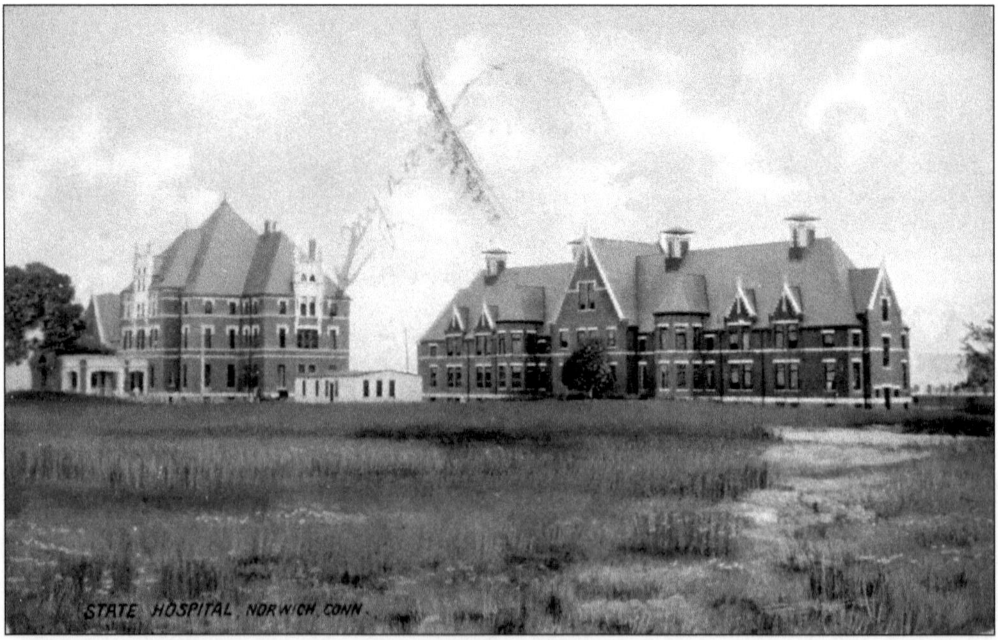

This 1910 postcard featuring the Administration Building (left) and Ward A North (right) also shows the continued use of the temporary office building while future wards and offices were being completed. The front of the postcard is pictured above, with a hand-drawn arrow pointing to a window on the third floor accompanied by the words "My room." A patient who was in Center Hospital on the third floor sent this card to a loved one. The writing on the back, shown below, suggests a quirky sense of humor about being an inpatient at a mental hospital: "Oh you Lunatic, I am thinking of you constantly, Sweetheart. I never thought I'd miss you as I do! How is the kid. M.G.H." (Both, author's collection.)

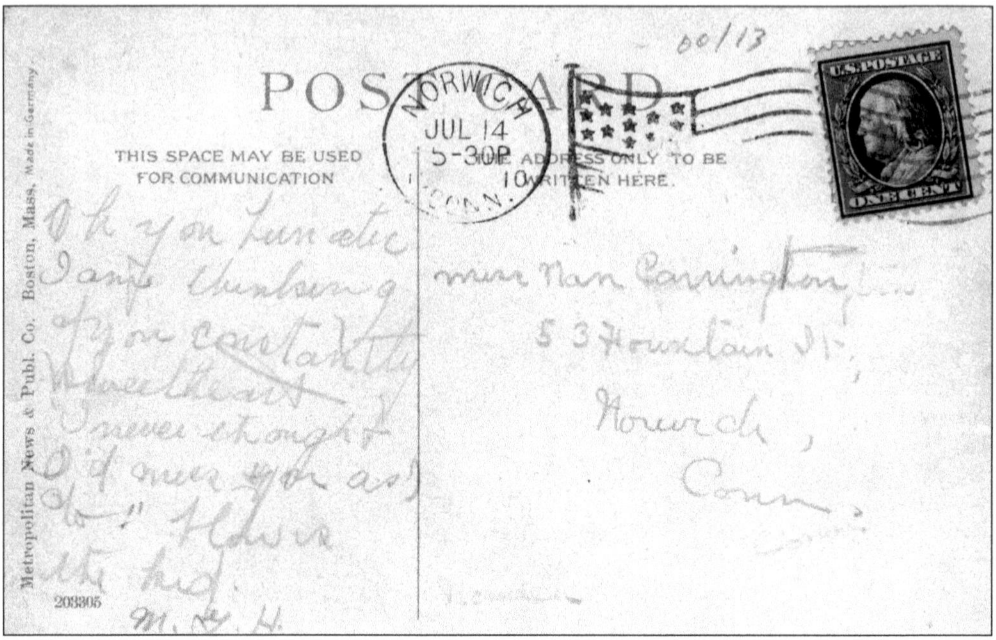

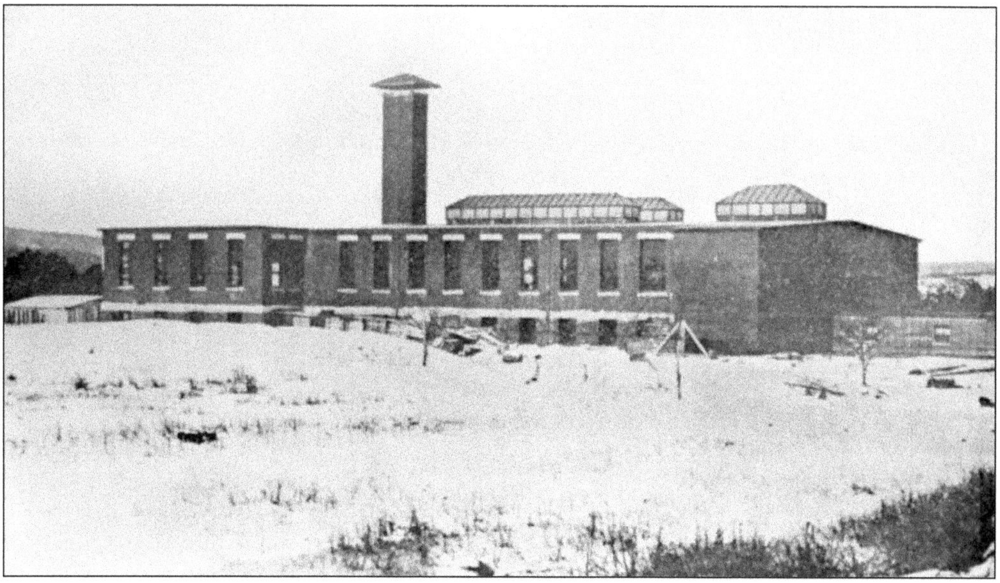

The first of the industrial buildings to be completed by 1906 were the hospital's permanent kitchen (above) and laundry (below). The large one-story kitchen occupied a central position between the wings of the ward buildings. The laundry building also occupied a central position and sat to the rear of the kitchen. The second story of the laundry building was occupied by sleeping rooms for 16 laundry employees. (Both, courtesy of Connecticut State Library.)

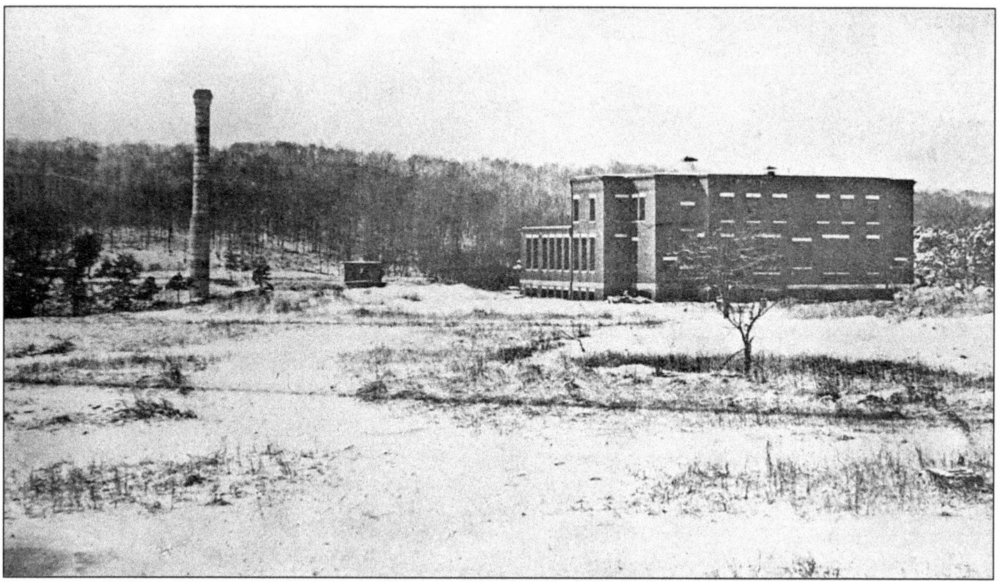

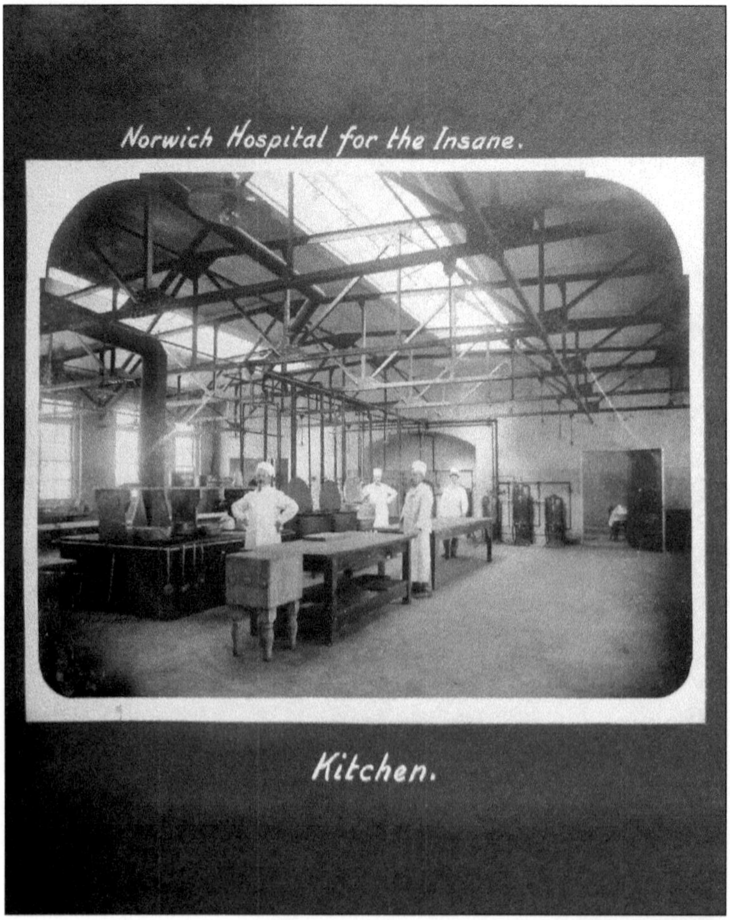

The main kitchen, pictured here in 1904, is where meals for 1,100 patients (as of 1915) and hundreds of hospital employees, the majority of whom lived on campus, were prepared. Most of the hospital's food was grown and raised on the grounds, with all cooking and baking done on the premises. An employee dining room was also housed in the main kitchen in addition to a scullery and a room for the cooks' daily stores. Included food and housing were some of the incentives to attract people to take jobs at the hospital for comparatively long hours and low wages. (Courtesy of Connecticut State Library.)

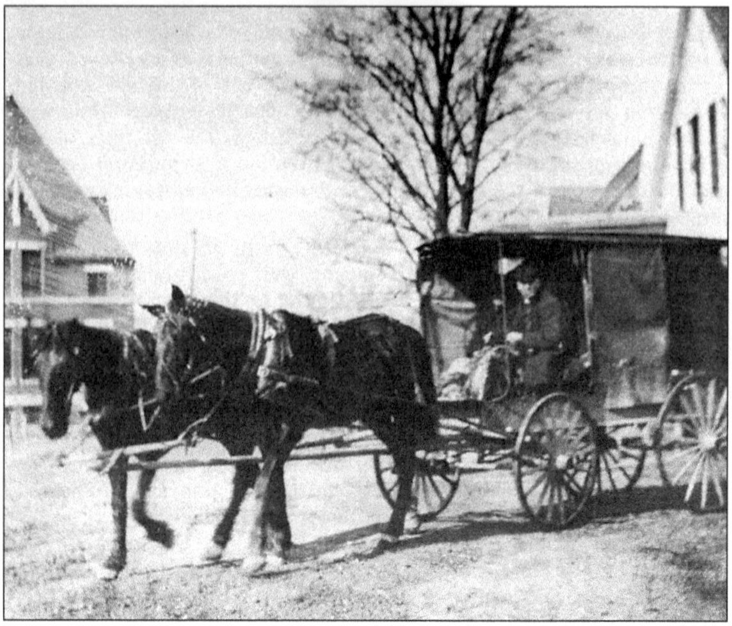

In the early 1900s, milk was delivered by horse and carriage to the main campus from the hospital's dairy farm. Milk was a staple in the kitchen and on the wards. Norwich Hospital for the Insane had its own horse barn for the breeding, raising, and care of horses. Horses worked alongside men plowing fields, planting crops, and distributing goods throughout the hospital grounds. (Author's collection.)

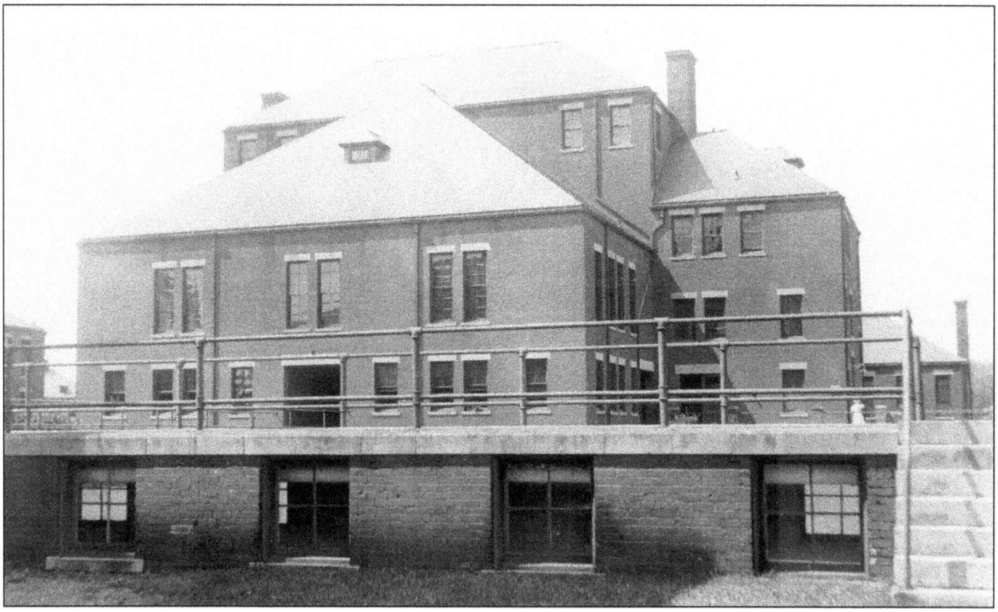

The amusement hall building adjoining the main kitchen was completed in 1912. Prior to the completion of this building, the hospital was only able to provide meager entertainment for its patients on the wards, in basement rooms, and in the Administration Building. Dr. Pollock repeatedly appealed to the General Assembly about the dire need for amusements for patients, emphasizing their importance as an aid to recovery. The amusement hall building contained a large dining room with a 600-person seating capacity, a social room/dance hall (which would later serve as a roller-skating rink), and a large auditorium for plays, musical concerts, meetings, religious services, and holiday celebrations. The auditorium comfortably seated 850. Both photographs are from 1931. (Both, courtesy of Preston Historical Society.)

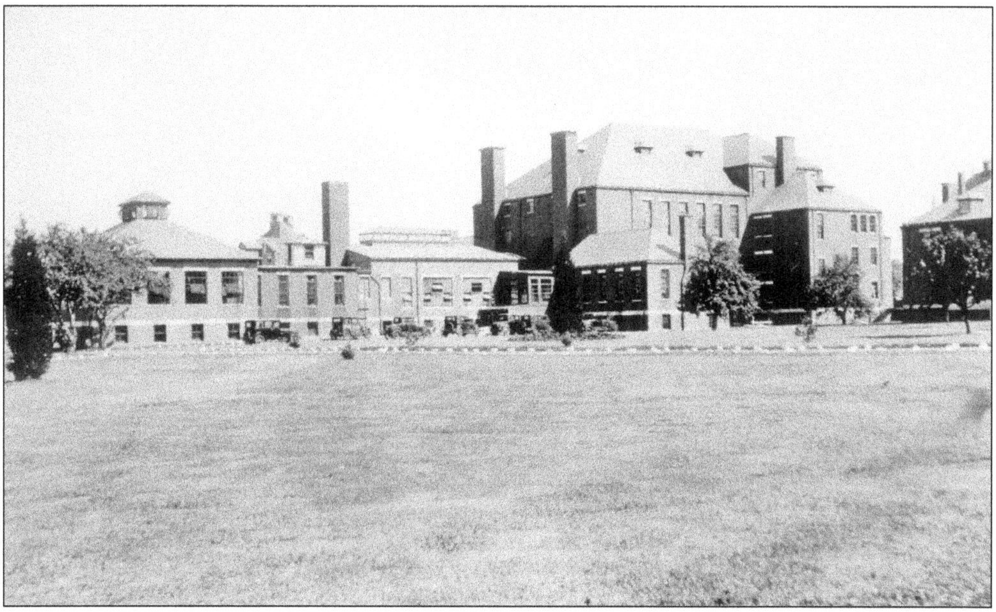

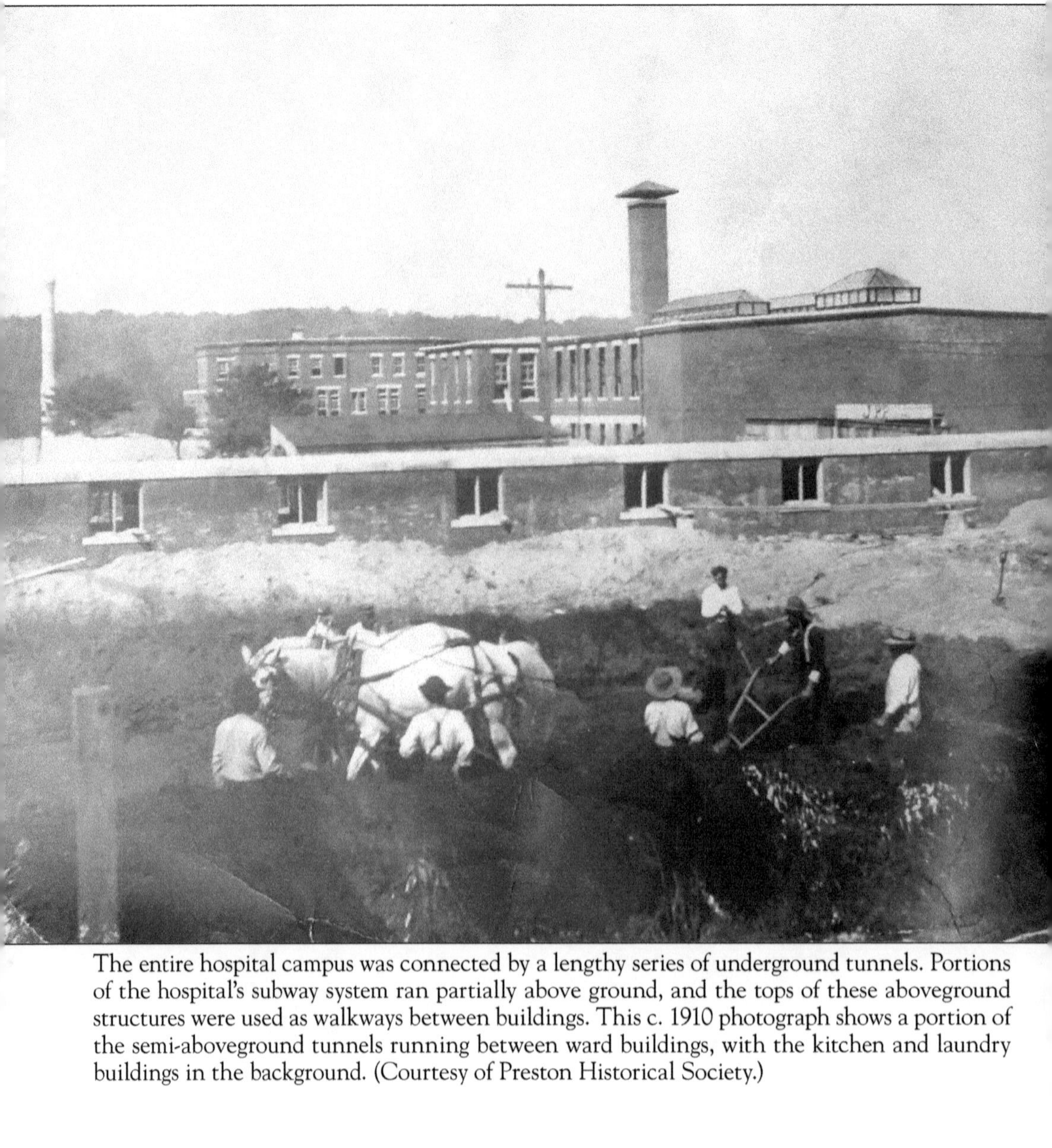

The entire hospital campus was connected by a lengthy series of underground tunnels. Portions of the hospital's subway system ran partially above ground, and the tops of these aboveground structures were used as walkways between buildings. This c. 1910 photograph shows a portion of the semi-aboveground tunnels running between ward buildings, with the kitchen and laundry buildings in the background. (Courtesy of Preston Historical Society.)

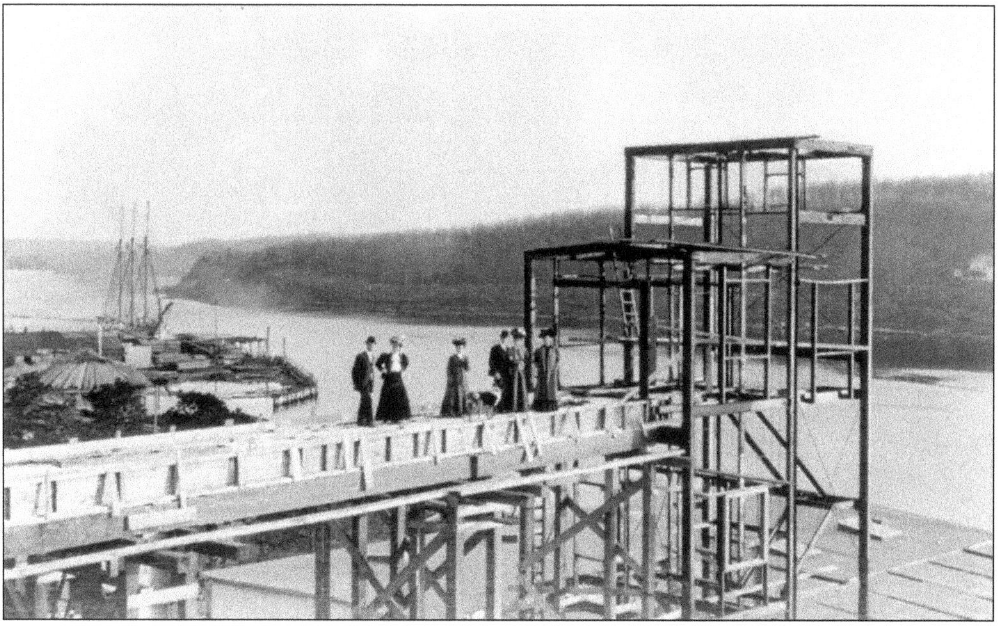

The hospital's main subway tunnel ran 977 feet in a straight line from the Administration Building at the front of the campus to the permanent powerhouse at the rear. The powerhouse was situated along a bank of the Thames River and adjacent to the tracks of the New York, New Haven & Hartford Railroad. This convenient location on the river was one of the key factors in this site being chosen for a second state hospital. Goods could be easily delivered and received by train and boat. A 108-foot-long bridge connected the powerhouse to the campus tunnel system. (Both, courtesy of Preston Historical Society.)

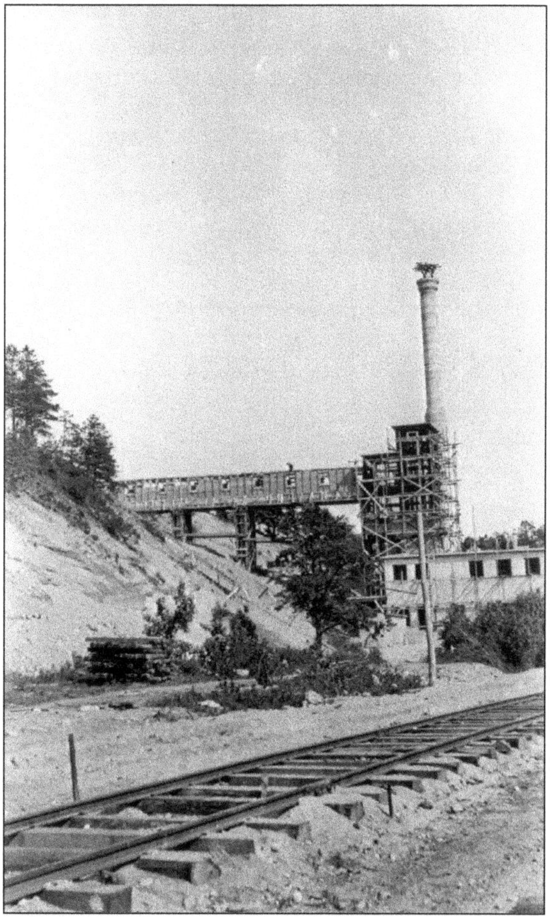

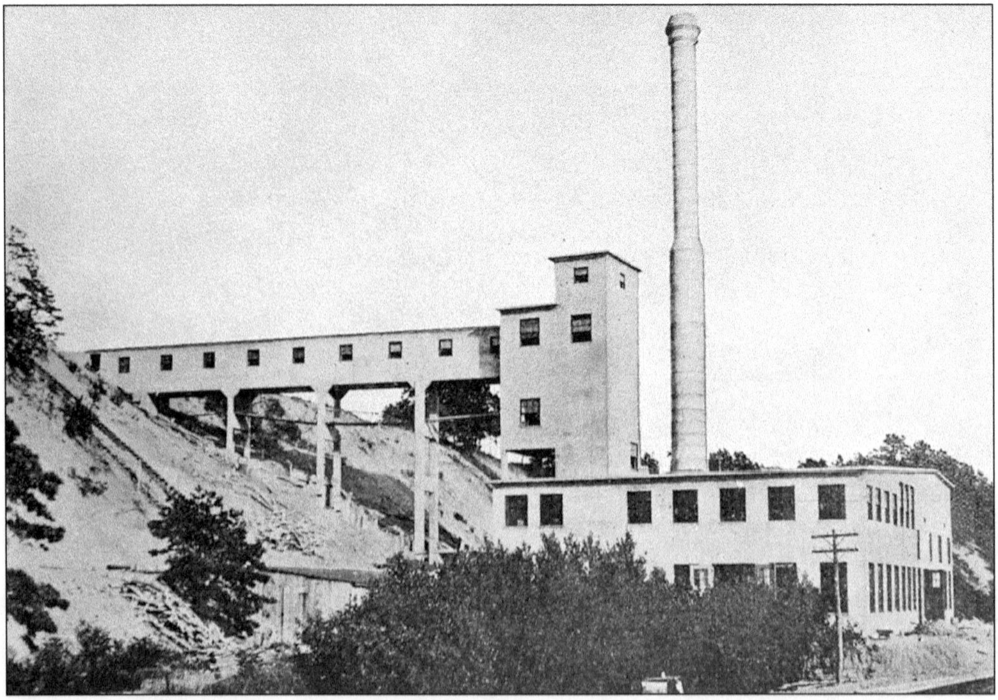

The completed powerhouse and connecting bridge are shown above in 1906. The powerhouse's smokestack rose 150 feet, with an internal diameter of six feet. The powerhouse cared for all the hospital's electrical, heating, and hot water needs. An opposite view of the powerhouse is shown below in 1931. The lower portion of the structure had a large storage room for the reception of freight from trains on the adjacent tracks. The powerhouse was equipped with an electric freight elevator capable of lifting two tons to carry goods delivered by boat and train up to the level of the tunnel for easy distribution throughout the hospital buildings. (Above, courtesy of Connecticut State Library; below, courtesy of Preston Historical Society.)

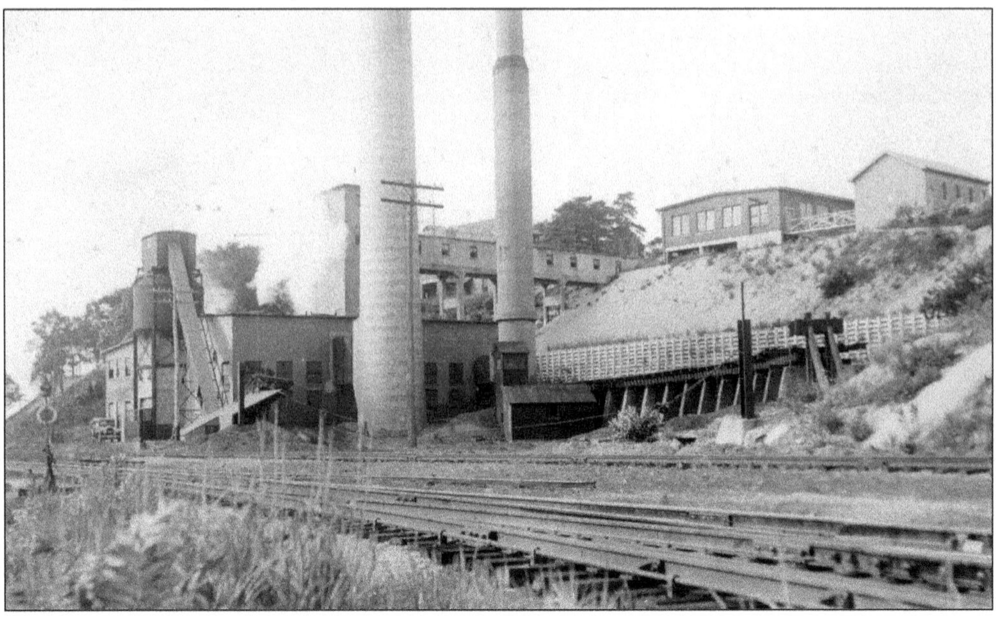

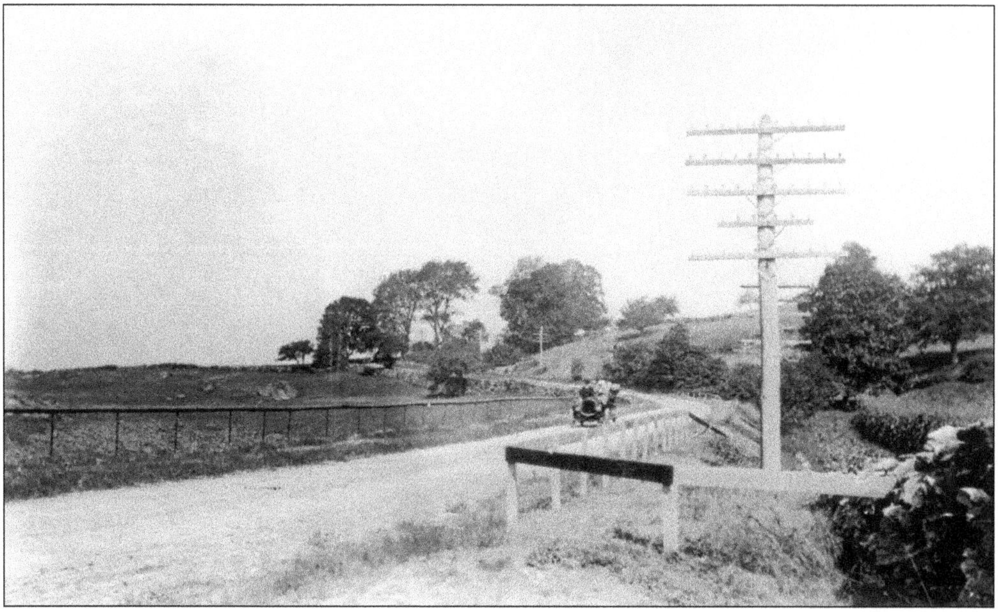

Route 12, immediately north of the Norwich State Hospital grounds, is shown here in 1910. The hill on the right in the rear would later become home to physician and attendant residences and additional ward buildings as the hospital expanded. (Courtesy of Preston Historical Society.)

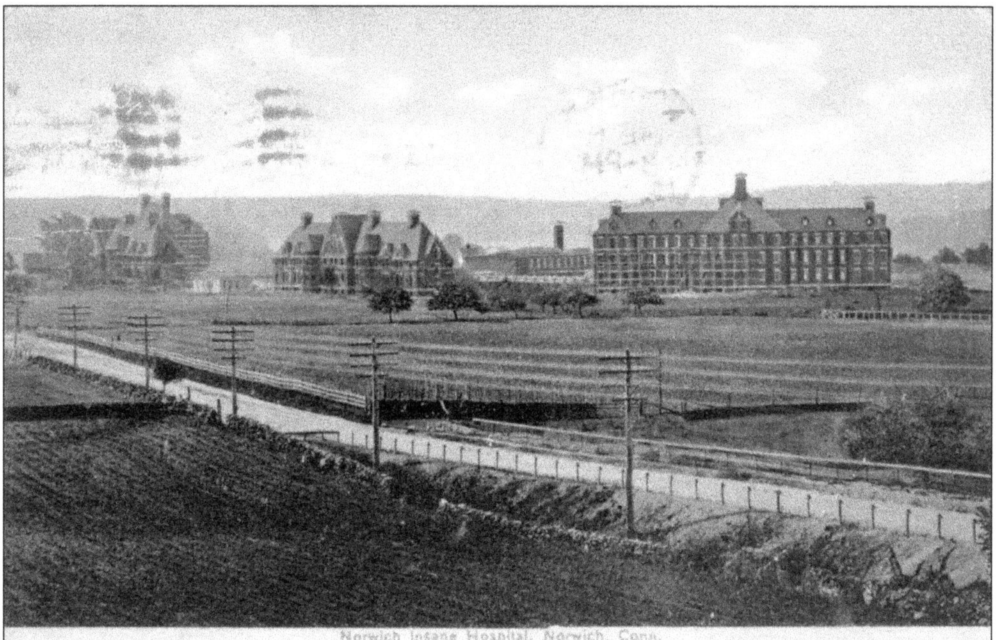

This postcard from 1907 provides a southern view of the first of Norwich State Hospital's ward buildings and Route 12, which was a dirt road lined with telegraph poles. (Author's collection.)

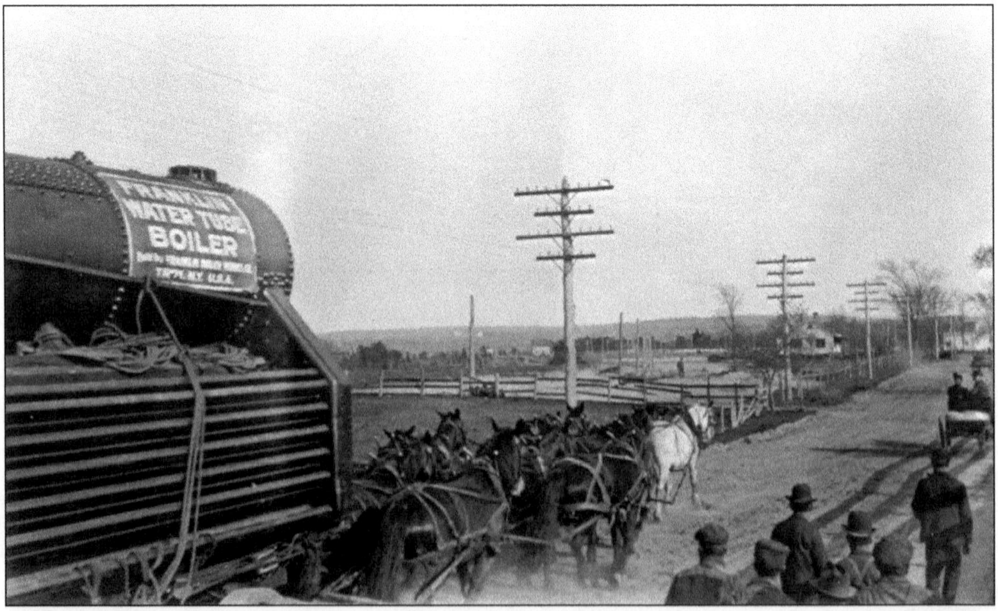

This c. 1910 photograph shows a team of horses and men transporting a new water boiler down the dirt Route 12 to the Norwich Hospital for the Insane. (Courtesy of Preston Historical Society.)

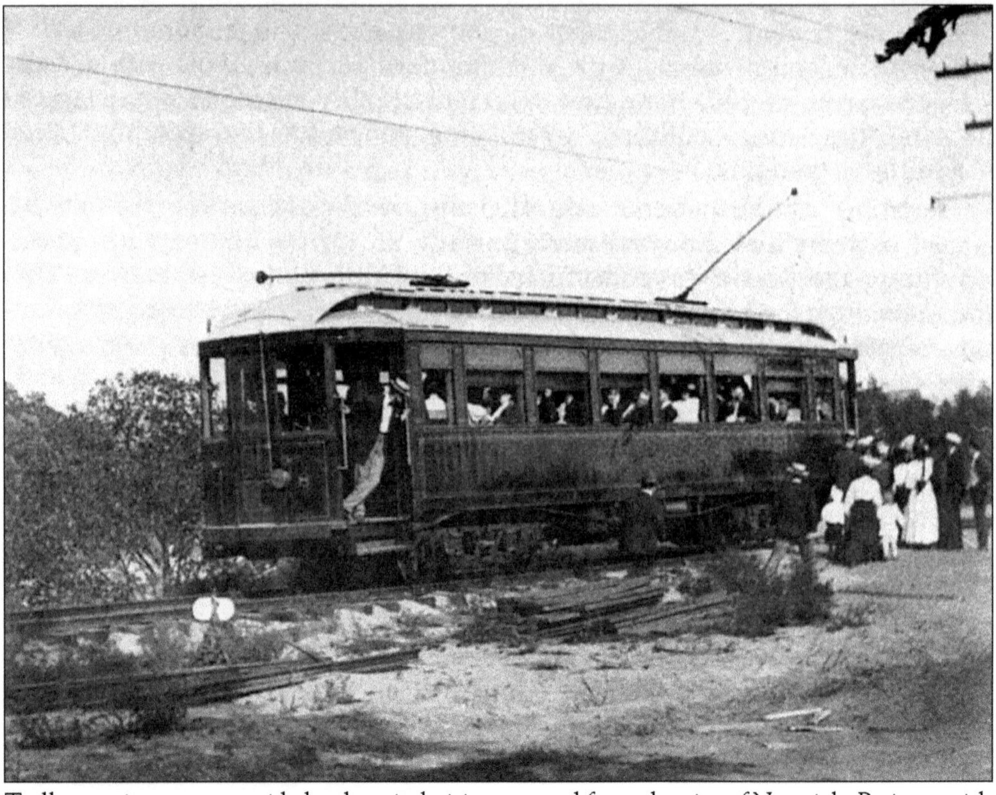

Trolley services were provided to hospital visitors to and from the city of Norwich. Patients with grounds privileges also used the trolley to spend afternoons shopping in and visiting Norwich. (Author's collection.)

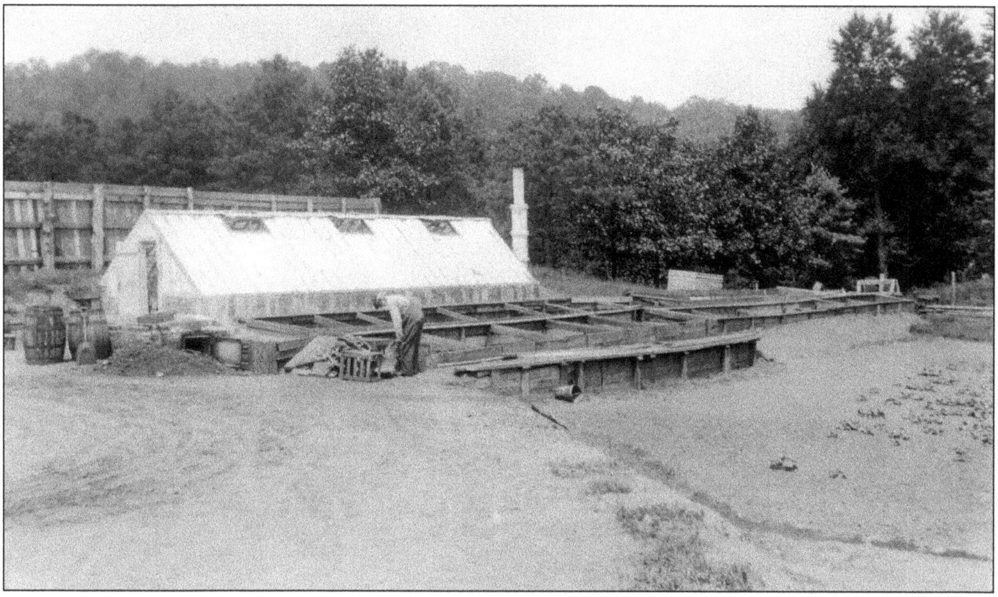

Norwich Hospital for the Insane's farmland had over 200 acres devoted to the growing of vegetables and fruits and the raising and slaughtering of hogs, turkeys, chicken, and cattle. A vegetable greenhouse is shown above, and the slaughterhouse is pictured below; both photographs were taken in 1931. Cows provided fresh milk for the patients and staff. The milk was pasteurized onsite in the hospital's own dairy farm. Nearly all of the ingredients for meals came directly from the hospital's farm. This type of self-sufficiency was characteristic of most mental hospitals around this time. State hospitals, Norwich included, were often referred to as "self-contained cities." (Both, courtesy of Preston Historical Society.)

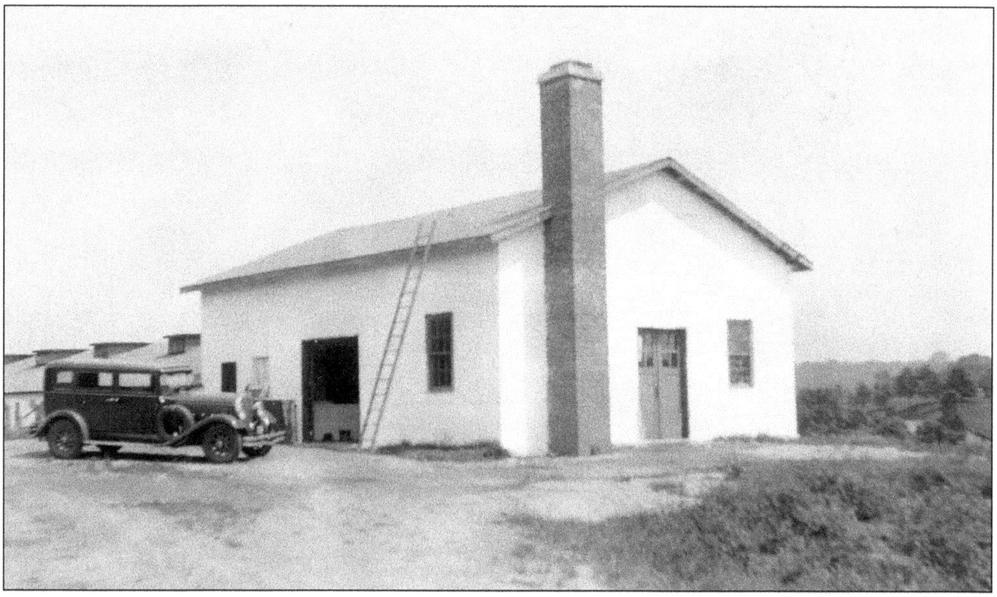

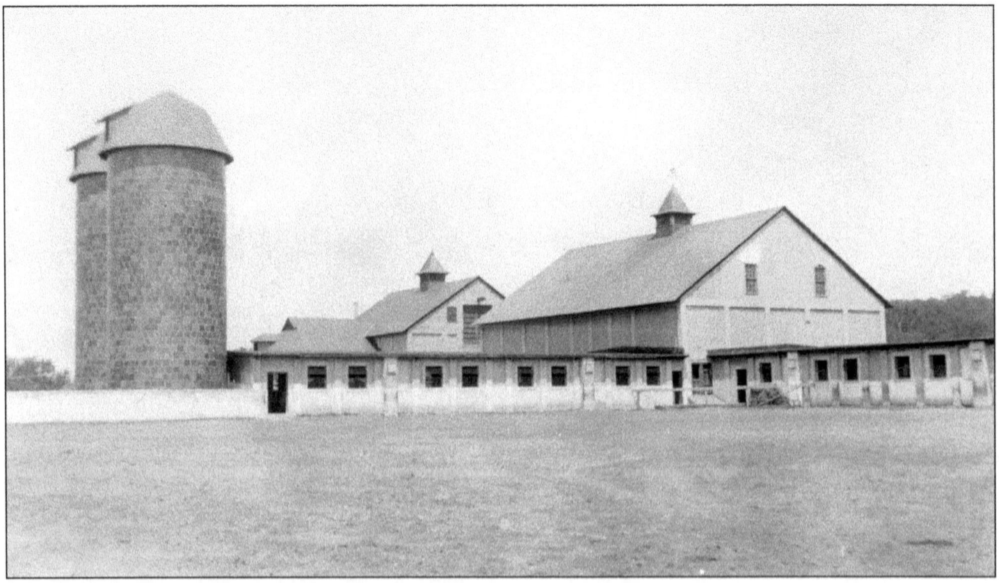

By 1930, the hospital was booming with 2,400 patients. In order to feed such a large number, the hospital's farm provided an impressive eight and a half barrels of flour from the granaries, 1,100 pounds of meat from the slaughterhouse, 1,200 to 1,800 quarts of milk and 85 pounds of butter from the dairies, 12 to 13 bushels of potatoes from the scullery, and at least 62 pounds of coffee and 30 pounds of tea on a daily basis. The cow barn and its silos are pictured above in 1931. Below is a 1904 view from inside the cow barn. (Above, courtesy of Preston Historical Society; below, courtesy of Connecticut State Library.)

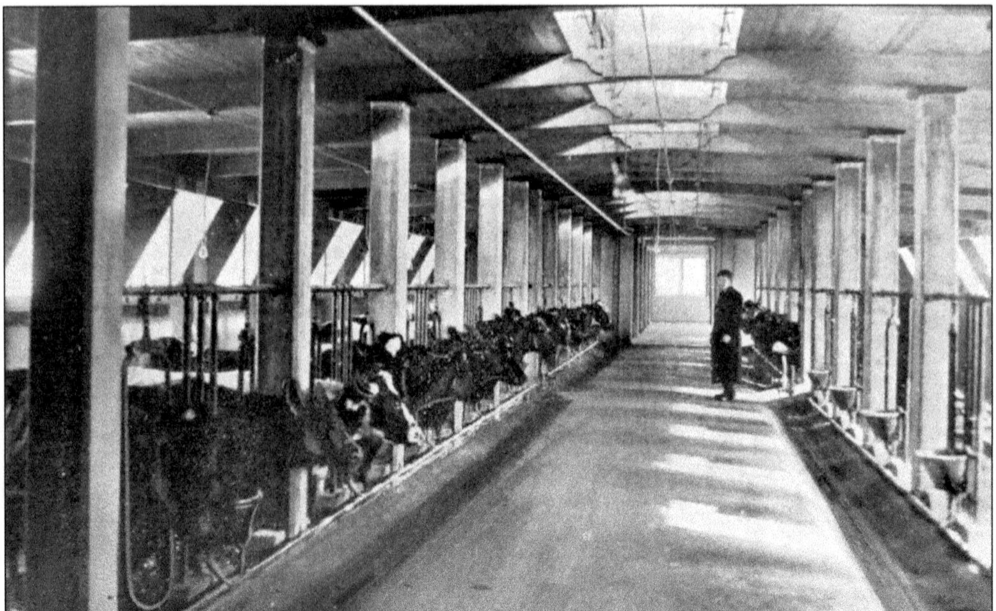

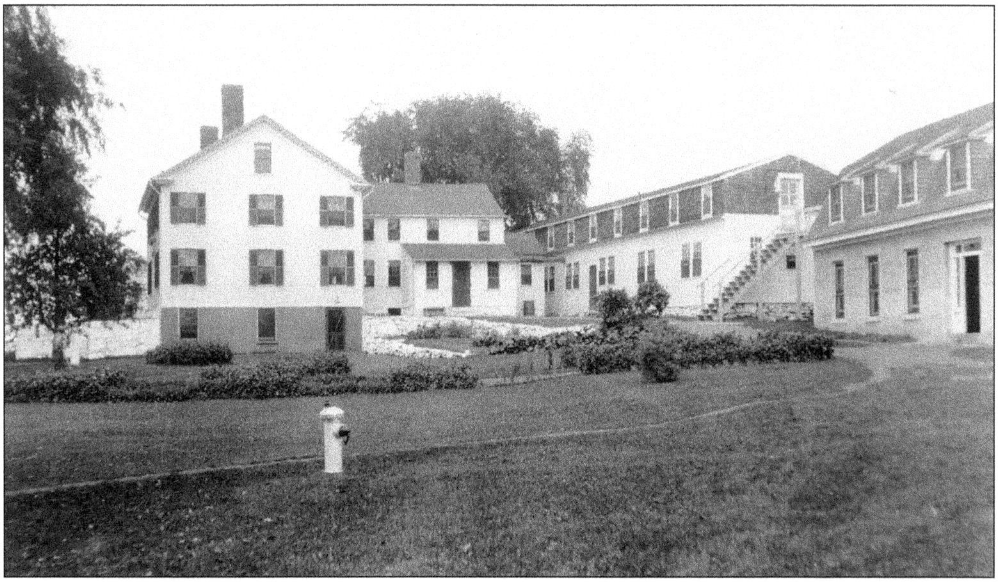

In 1910, Dr. Pollock advocated to the General Assembly for the establishment of a Hospital Farm for Inebriates. The hospital had an unusually large number of patients who were not "insane" but were found to be dipsomaniacs. Dr. Pollock felt that dipsomaniacs did not belong with the general hospital population and would benefit from a separately established farm for their recovery. The General Assembly ignored his repeated requests until 1916, when the Hospital Farm for Inebriates was finally established. The site chosen for the "Inebriate Farm" was the 100-acre Gallup Farm, two and a half miles east of the main hospital. The farm's buildings consisted of a large house with an adjoining shed. This shed was remodeled to contain a kitchen, serving room, and dining room while the second story was made into a very comfortable dormitory (at center above). An additional 20 by 30 foot building was erected on the south end of the first dormitory building, extending the dining room capacity to 100 and the dormitory to 36 (below). (Both, courtesy of Preston Historical Society.)

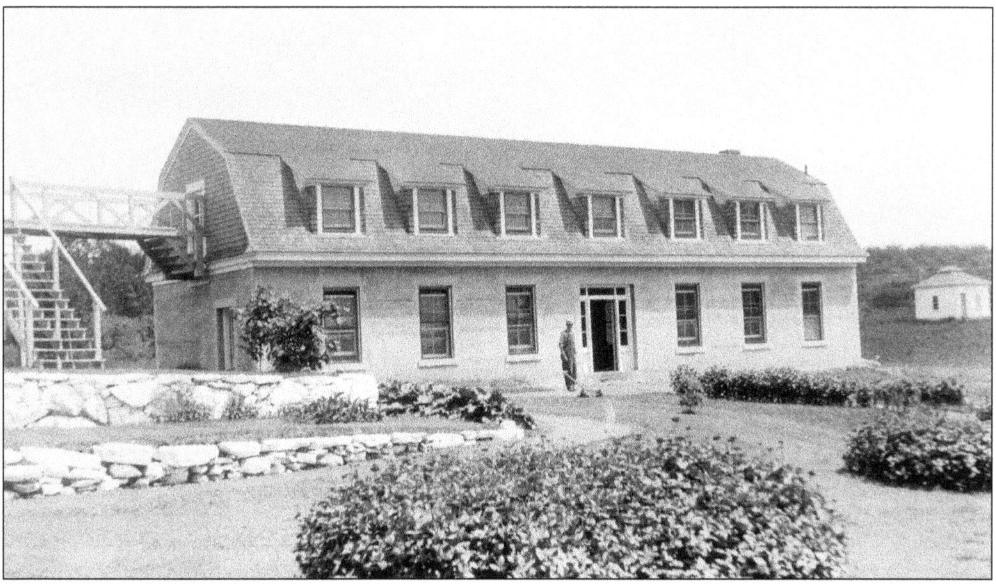

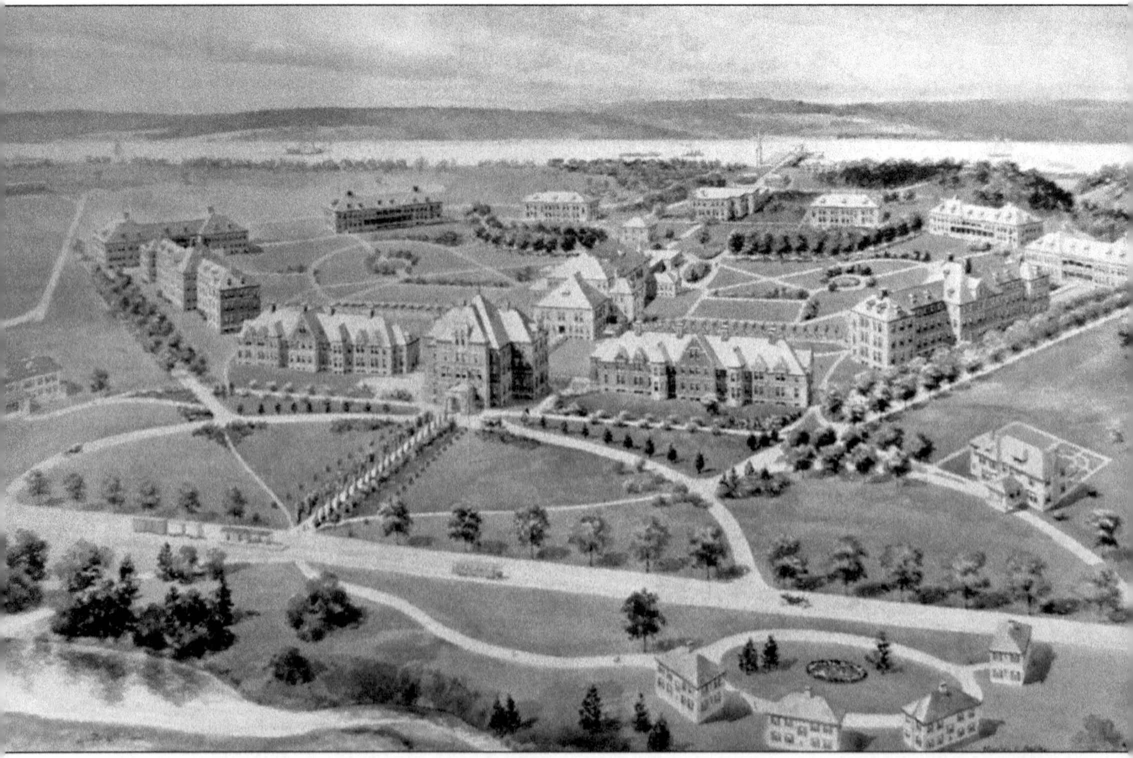

This artist's aerial view depicts the completed hospital's symmetrical campus as of 1915. The patient census in that year was 1,030. Overcrowding beyond the limits of comfort and safety would again prevail, and the hospital would again find itself appealing to the General Assembly for funding to construct additional ward buildings to accommodate the steady increase. (Courtesy of Connecticut State Library.)

Two

Institutional Ups and Downs

Dr. Henry Pollock left Norwich Hospital for the Insane in 1916 to accept the position as superintendent of the Massachusetts Homeopathic Hospital in Boston. He continued to affiliate with Norwich Hospital for the Insane, serving as a consultant until 1940. Dr. Pollock's successors shared his wishes for mentally ill persons to be respected and treated with dignity. They believed the word "insane" brought public shame and disgrace to the patients and their families and to the hospital. They continued to advocate for its elimination from the hospital's name. They wanted Connecticut to be proud of her state institutions. Sadly, Dr. Pollock did not see this effort come to fruition during his superintendence. Three years after his departure for Boston, the hospital's name was finally changed to Norwich State Hospital.

Dr. Pollock's successor, Dr. Franklin S. Wilcox, was severely criticized for publicly stating his belief that insane persons with no hope of recovery should be put to death if, after 15 to 20 years of expert observation, the illness did not improve. Even for a time when mental illness was often seen as shameful and those stricken were not treated equally in the community, his comments caused a public outrage. Former Connecticut governor Everett Lake was shaken by the comments and stated that such treatment "is quite out of harmony with our social views and absolutely contrary to our established public policy." Dr. Wilcox submitted his resignation in 1928 following these criticisms and an investigation of the Inebriate Farm. He declined to state a public reason for his departure.

Patient numbers continued to climb and Norwich State Hospital went through another growth spurt by 1930 with the addition of more ward buildings and employee housing. Amidst this growth, the hospital suffered more ups and downs. Epidemics of dysentery (which claimed at least 12 patient lives), deplorable ward conditions, mistreatment of patients, poor hospital management, and lack of accreditation by the American Psychiatric Association led to more hurdles Norwich State Hospital would have to overcome.

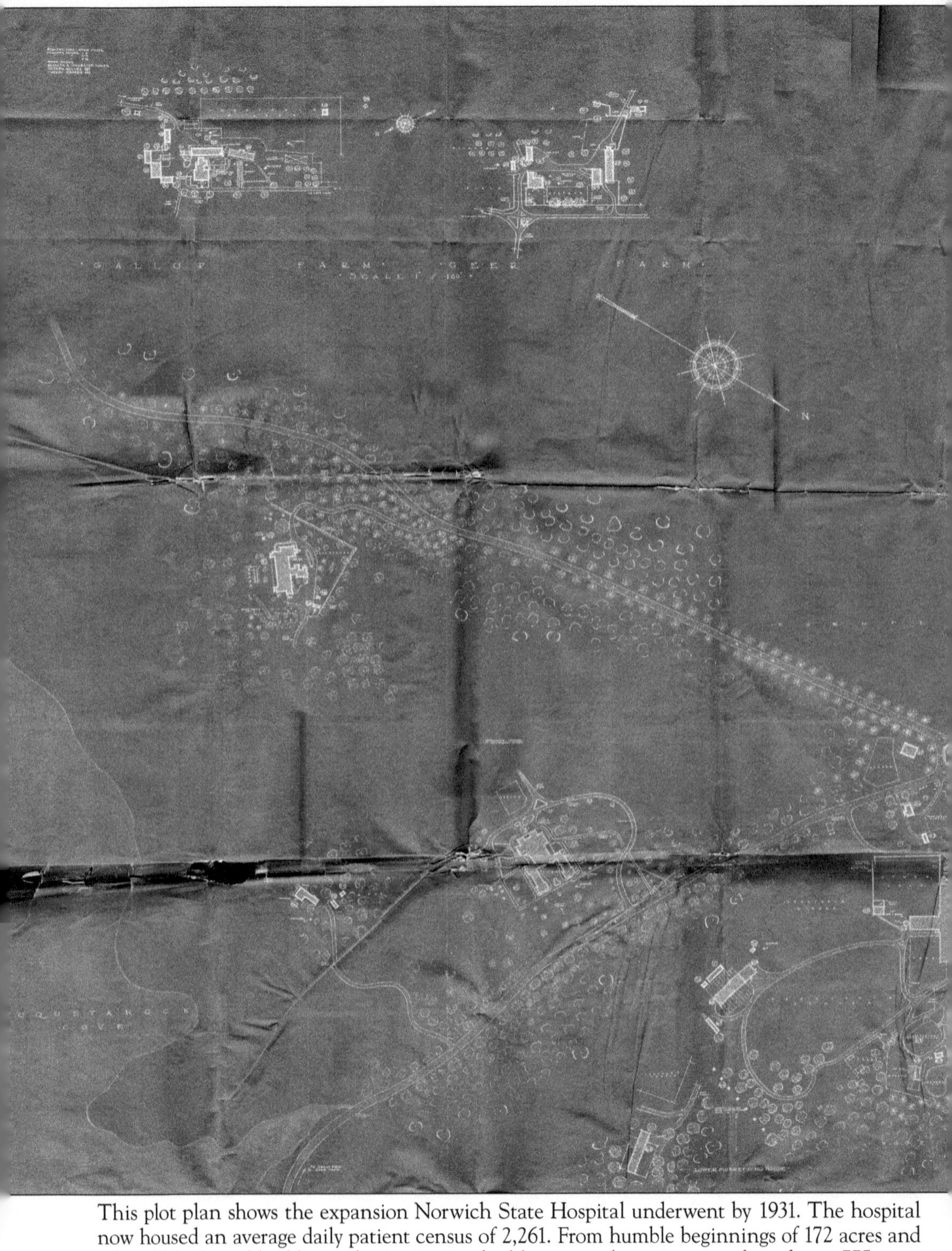

This plot plan shows the expansion Norwich State Hospital underwent by 1931. The hospital now housed an average daily patient census of 2,261. From humble beginnings of 172 acres and a handful of ward buildings, the institution had become a booming complex of over 775 acres and over 35 buildings. These included the Administration Building, over 20 ward buildings for

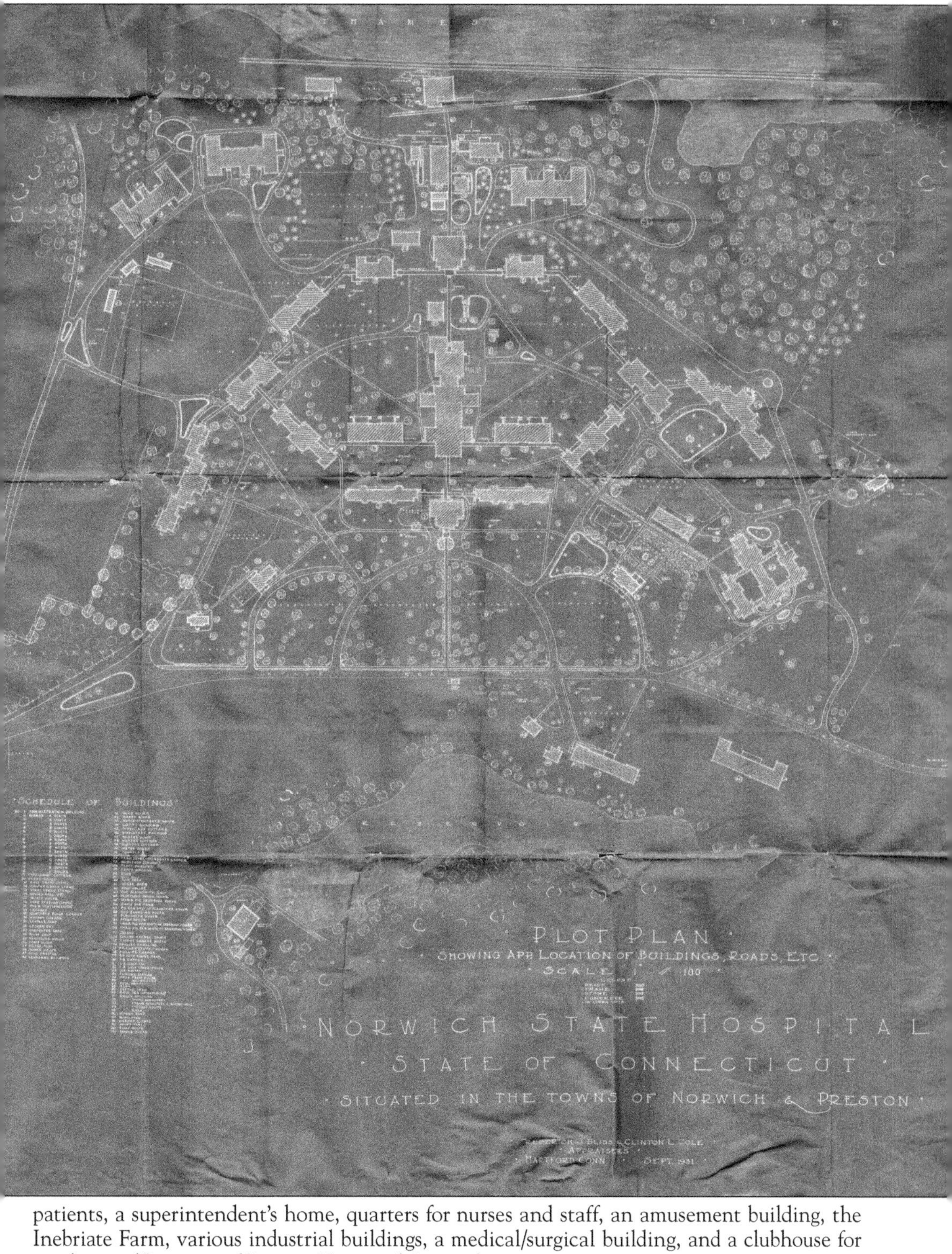
SCHEDULE OF BUILDINGS
PLOT PLAN
SHOWING APP LOCATION OF BUILDINGS, ROADS, ETC.
NORWICH STATE HOSPITAL
STATE OF CONNECTICUT
SITUATED IN THE TOWNS OF NORWICH & PRESTON

patients, a superintendent's home, quarters for nurses and staff, an amusement building, the Inebriate Farm, various industrial buildings, a medical/surgical building, and a clubhouse for employees. (Courtesy of Preston Historical Society.)

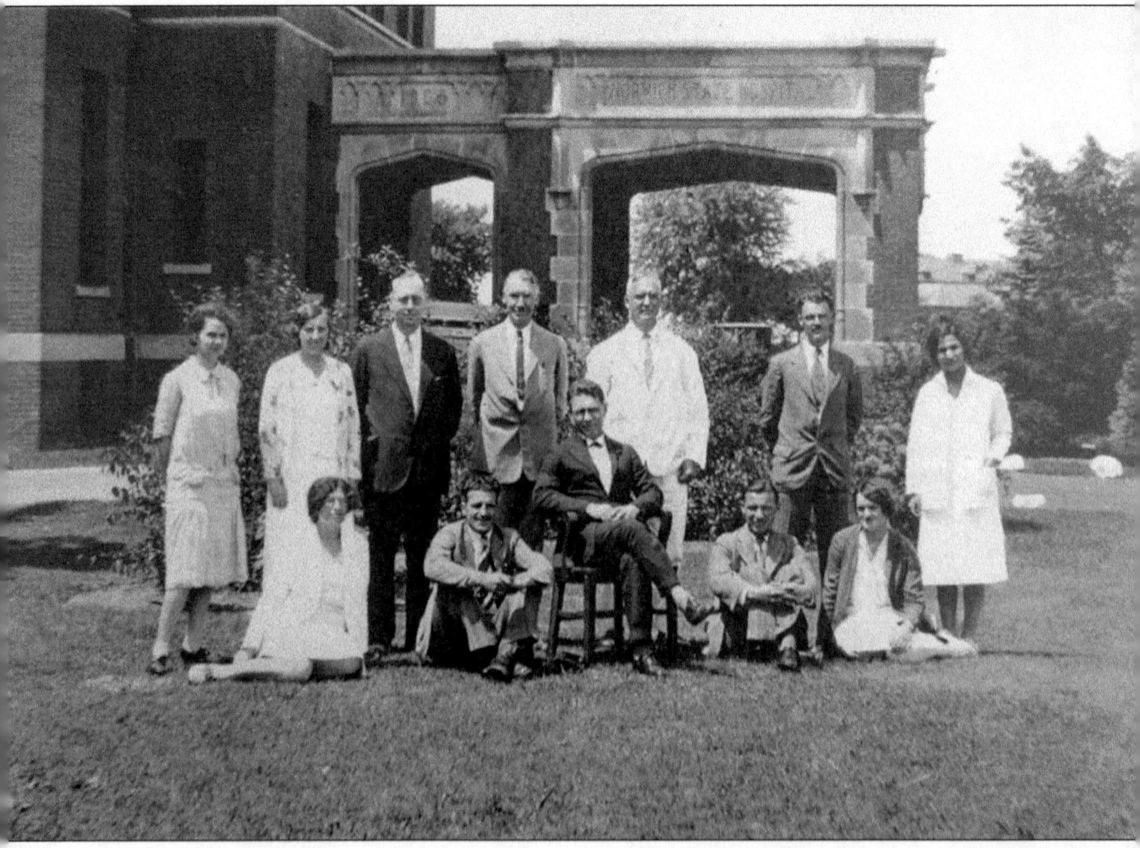

Dr. Elijah S. Burdsall, seated at center, appears in this 1930 photograph with his medical and clinical staff. Dr. Burdsall succeeded Dr. Wilcox in 1928 and then stepped down in 1934 to accept appointment as clinical director, as he desired to give more direct treatment to his patients. He left Norwich State Hospital in 1938. Dr. Chester Waterman was his successor. (Courtesy of Connecticut State Library.)

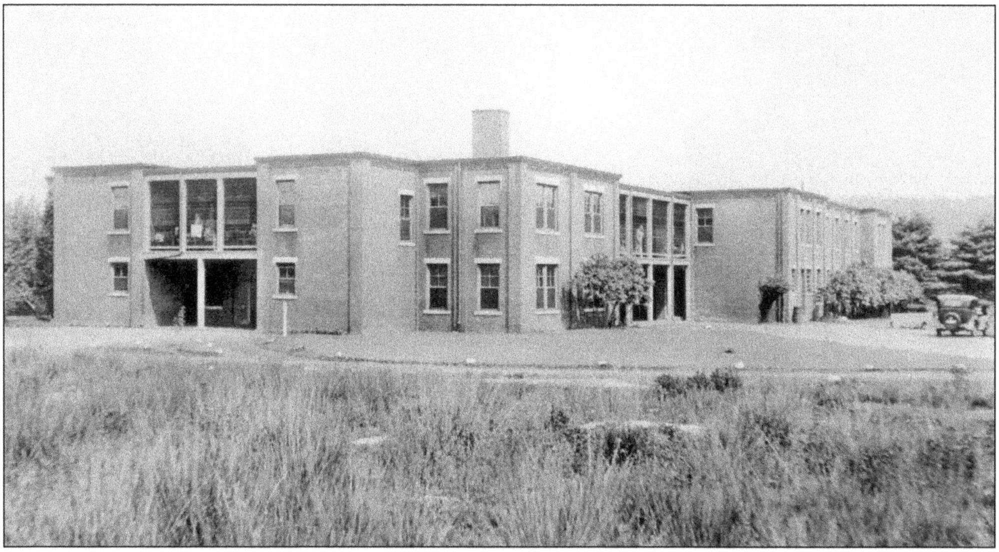

By 1934, the buildings of the Gallup Farm were so dilapidated that the hospital administration moved the Inebriate Farm into the old Farm Colony building (pictured above in 1931). The experiment of segregating dipsomaniacs from the general population of the state hospital initiated by Dr. Pollock in 1910 began to be seen as a failure by 1926. The hospital repeatedly defended accusations that bootleggers and drug peddlers had easy access to the farm's inmates and that inmates frequently escaped. Some farm inmates had secret liquor stashes and operated small stills in the woods adjacent to the farm. The Public Welfare Council investigated these complaints in 1937. Dr. Waterman concurred with the council's recommendation of shutting down the farm. After being called "absolutely useless" for curing drunkards in the media, "An Act Abolishing the State Farm for Inebriates" was signed by the governor on April 5, 1939. The closed Inebriate Farm is pictured below after 1950. (Above, courtesy of Preston Historical Society; below, courtesy of Brian Girasoli.)

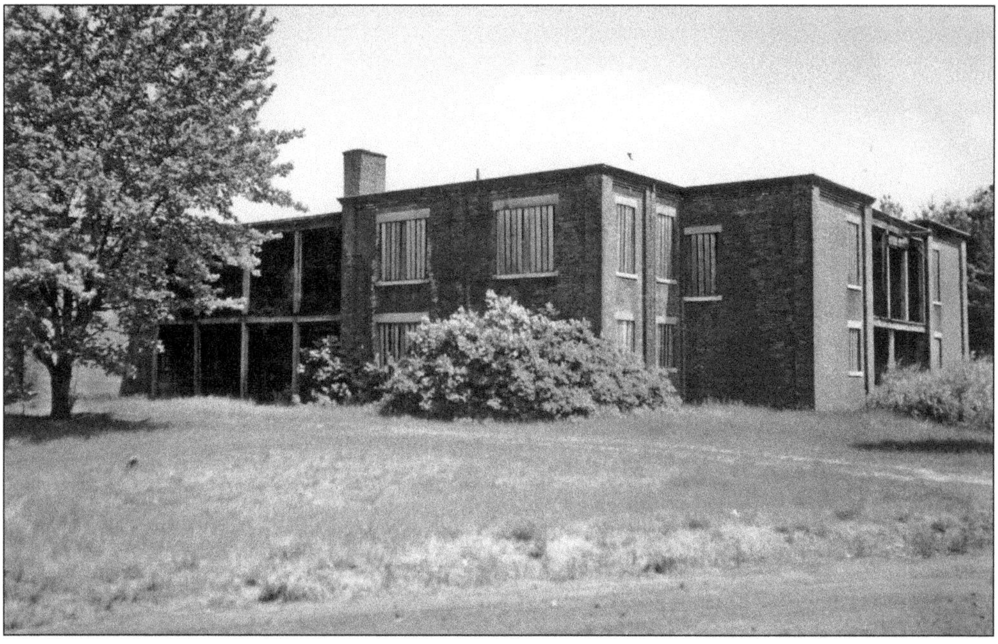

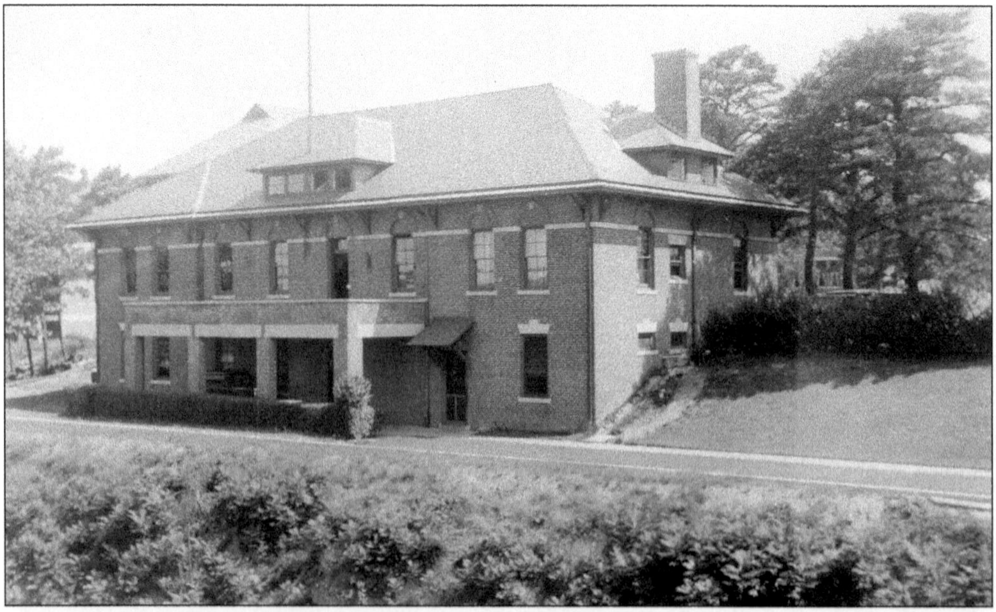

An innovative addition to the hospital, a recreational clubhouse for employees, was formally opened on November 26, 1913. During his superintendence, Dr. Pollock wanted to create a new incentive for his current employees and attract people seeking meaningful employment to the state hospital. Many hospital attendants were working an arduous 73.5 hours per week and spent an average of 14 hours per day in direct contact with their charges. Many lived on the wards. Dr. Pollock knew he could not retain good employees and expect them to perform at their best without a place for rest, relaxation, and rejuvenation. The clubhouse for employees was the first of its kind to be erected at a state hospital with a specific appropriation by a state legislature in the country. The clubhouse featured bowling alleys, a gymnasium, rooms for games and card playing, and a small store where refreshments could be purchased. It was not uncommon for an employee to have little left of his weekly salary after purchasing refreshments at the clubhouse. (Both, courtesy of Preston Historical Society.)

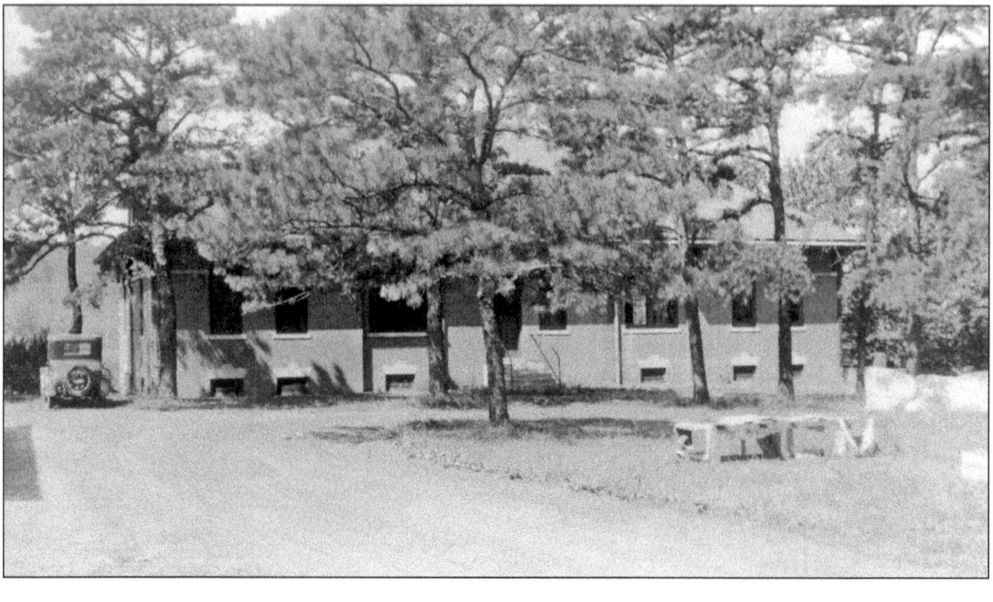

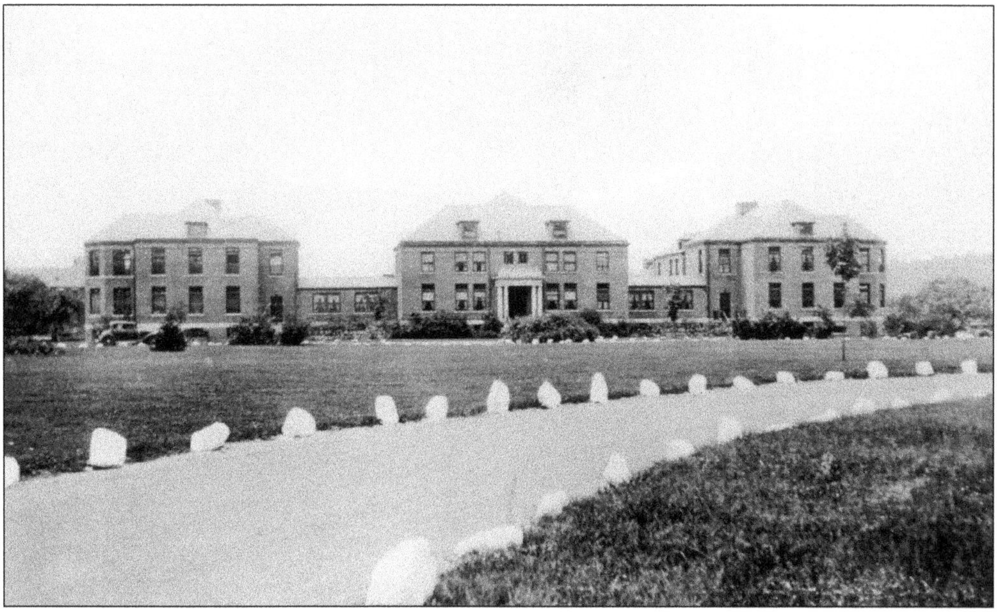

A reception hospital, originally called the Psychopathic Hospital, was opened for the reception and treatment of patients on July 5, 1921. It was later named for Norwich mayor, prominent banker, and president of the board of trustees Costello Lippitt. Lippitt served on the hospital's board from its inception in 1903 until his death in 1924. Medical and surgical services were provided here for patients and employees. Sterilizations, convulsive therapies, and prefrontal lobotomy procedures were also performed in this building. (Above, courtesy of Preston Historical Society; right, courtesy of Otis Library.)

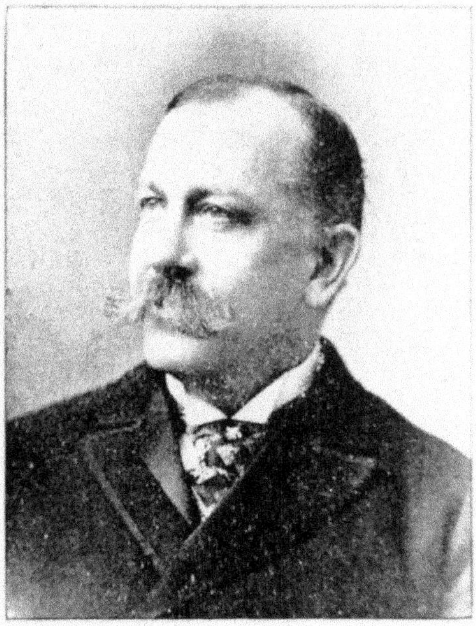

COSTELLO LIPPITT,
Treasurer Norwich Savings Society.

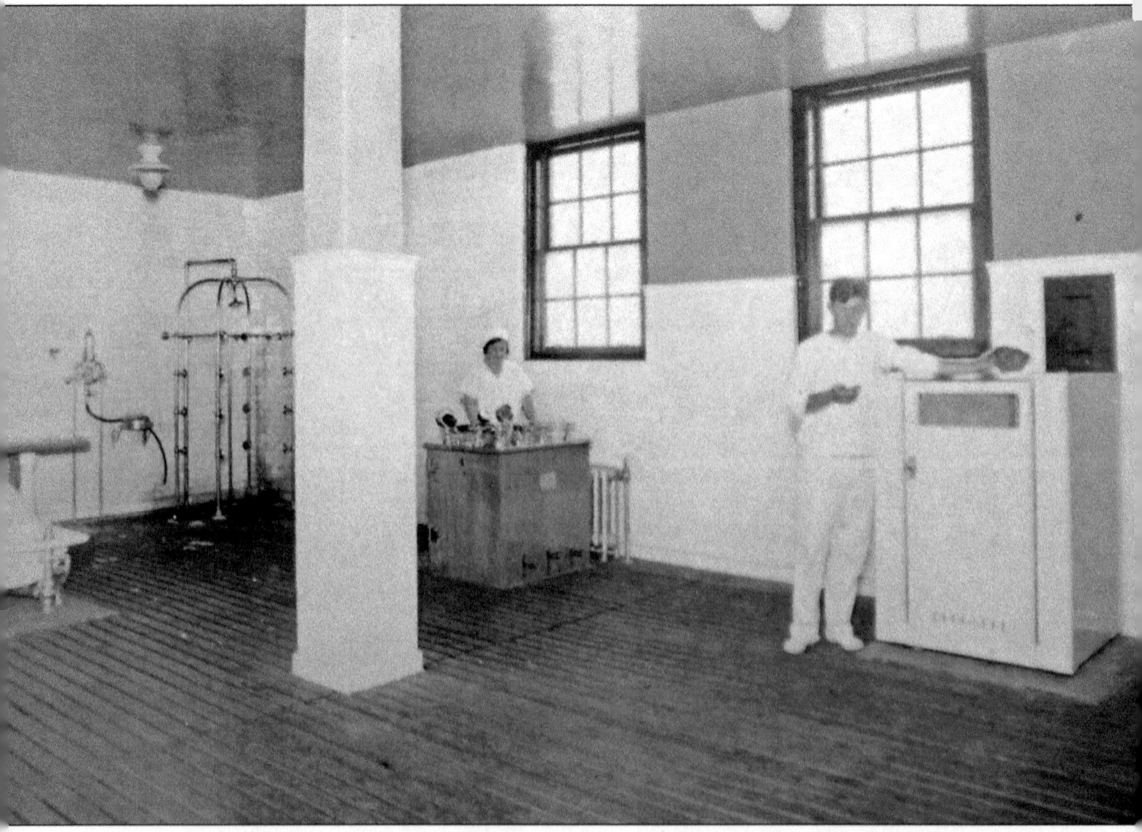

Beginning in 1936, convulsive treatments such as Metrazol were used with skepticism on a few select dementia praecox (now known as schizophrenia) patients. Shortly thereafter, insulin coma therapy was used in treating schizophrenic cases. Hospital superintendents during this time had serious doubts as to both treatments' effectiveness and safety. Metrazol shock therapy produced seizures so violent, a patient receiving the therapy often suffered fractures of the spine or dislocation of the shoulders and jaw. Metrazol shock and insulin coma therapies were completely discontinued and replaced with electro-convulsive therapies by 1942. Hydrotherapy units in the Lippitt Building, as pictured here around 1930, were favored over mechanical restraint by physicians for their calming effects on excited patients. Hydrotherapy patients were placed for long hours in a continuous bath in which staff regulated the water temperature. Patients were suspended in a canvas hammock inside the tub, often in their pajamas, with circulating water aimed to cool their temperament. Cold, wet sheet packs were also used to calm patients; however, they were used more as a threat of punishment against unruly types. Often, these punishments were not just idle threats. (Courtesy of Connecticut State Library.)

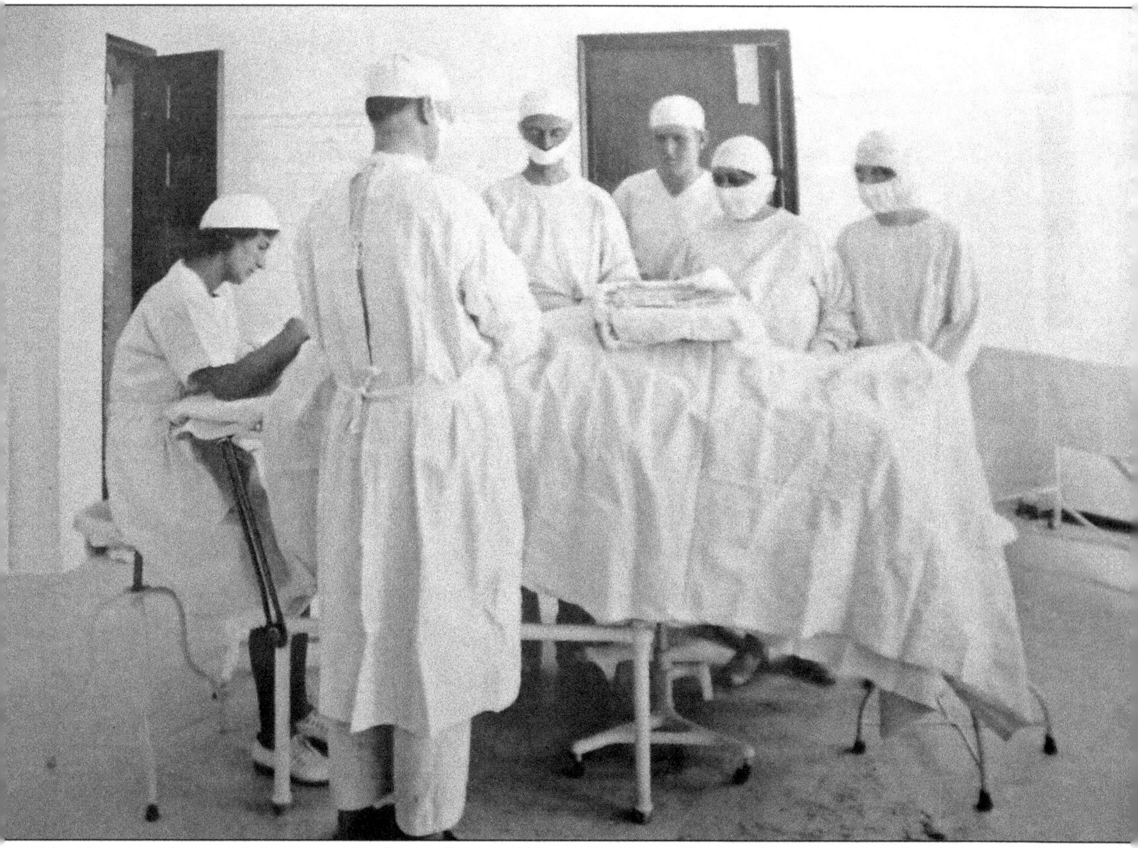

The first prefrontal lobotomy performed on a Norwich State Hospital patient was done at New Haven Hospital in 1946. All subsequent lobotomies were performed in the Lippitt Building's surgical rooms. By 1948, only four of the procedures had been performed. The board of trustees believed that NSH should have an active lobotomy program, trusting that the surgical benefits of lobotomy would raise discharge rates and ease overcrowding. NSH and its two sister state hospitals became part of the Connecticut Cooperative Lobotomy Study. Prominent neurosurgeon Dr. William Beecher Scoville, founder of the Department of Neurosurgery at Hartford Hospital in 1939, was one of the many surgeons to perform lobotomies on patients at NSH. Lobotomy procedures began to be phased out in the 1950s with the advent of new psychotropic drugs such as Thorazine and Haldol. By the 1950s, lobotomy procedures were seen as labor-intensive and not the hoped miracle cure for mental illness that had been hyped to the public. Thorazine produced what psychiatrists called a "chemical lobotomy," as the effects of the drug on a patient were similar to that of the operative procedure. (Courtesy of Connecticut State Library.)

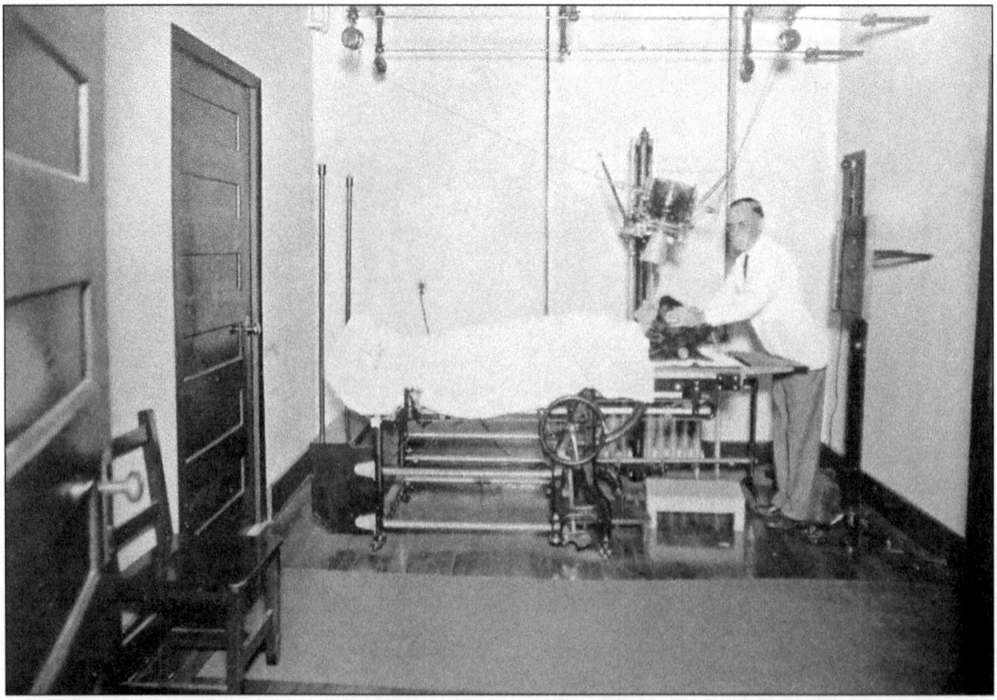

The Lippitt Building had state-of-the-art X-ray suites, which the hospital was very proud of. Hundreds of radiographic images were created each year to aid in diagnosing a large variety of medical problems. The hospital's administration strongly believed that no patient could be properly treated without a comprehensive physical examination upon admission to rule out the possibility of physical ailments contributing to their mental illness. (Above, courtesy of Connecticut State Library; below, courtesy of Lloyd Langhammer.)

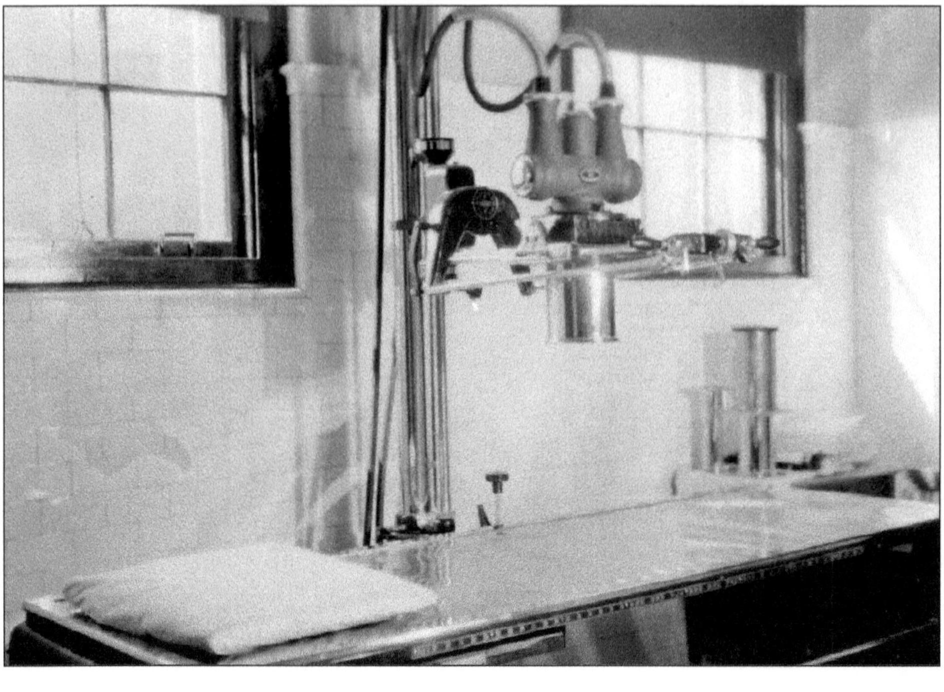

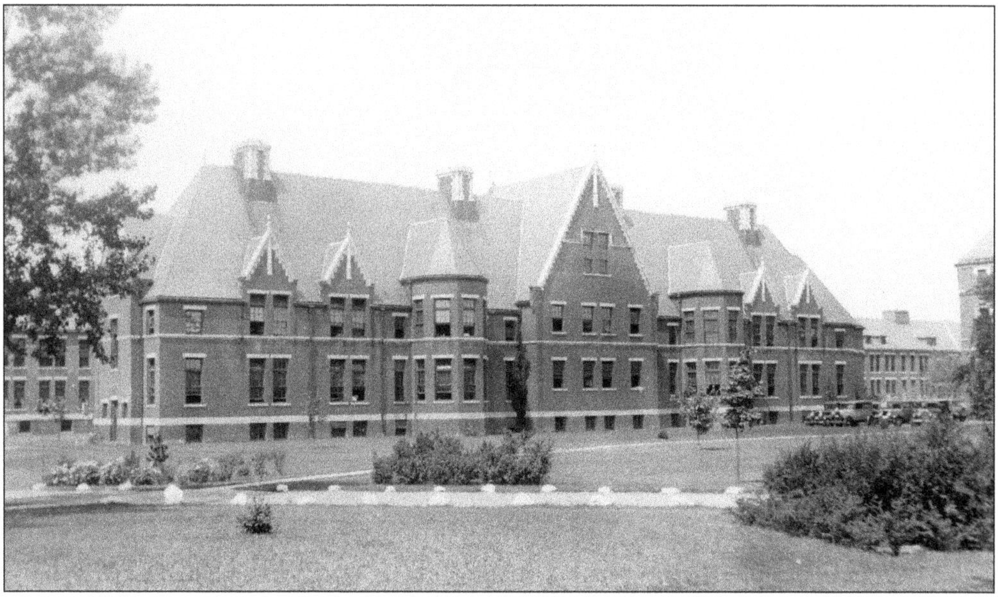

By 1930, Ward A South ceased its patient use and was attractively furnished and repurposed as housing for male employees. Male employees were relocated from Ward A South into a brand-new building across the street from the main campus in 1931. The uncompleted male employees' building is seen below that same year. In 1937, Ward A South was renovated and converted to house a class of patient that had been a recurring problem for the hospital since its inception: the state's criminally insane. (Both, courtesy of Preston Historical Society.)

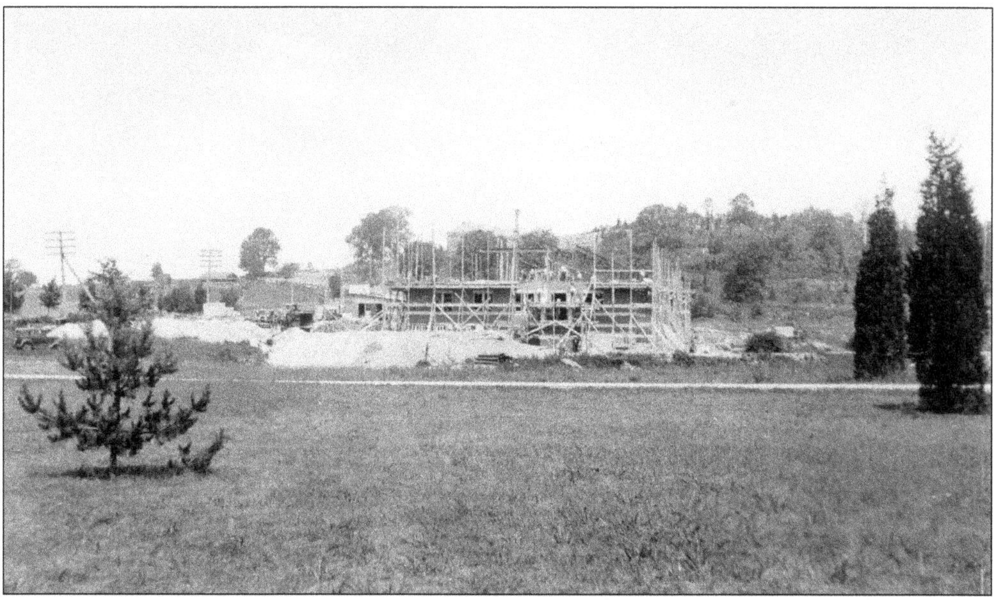

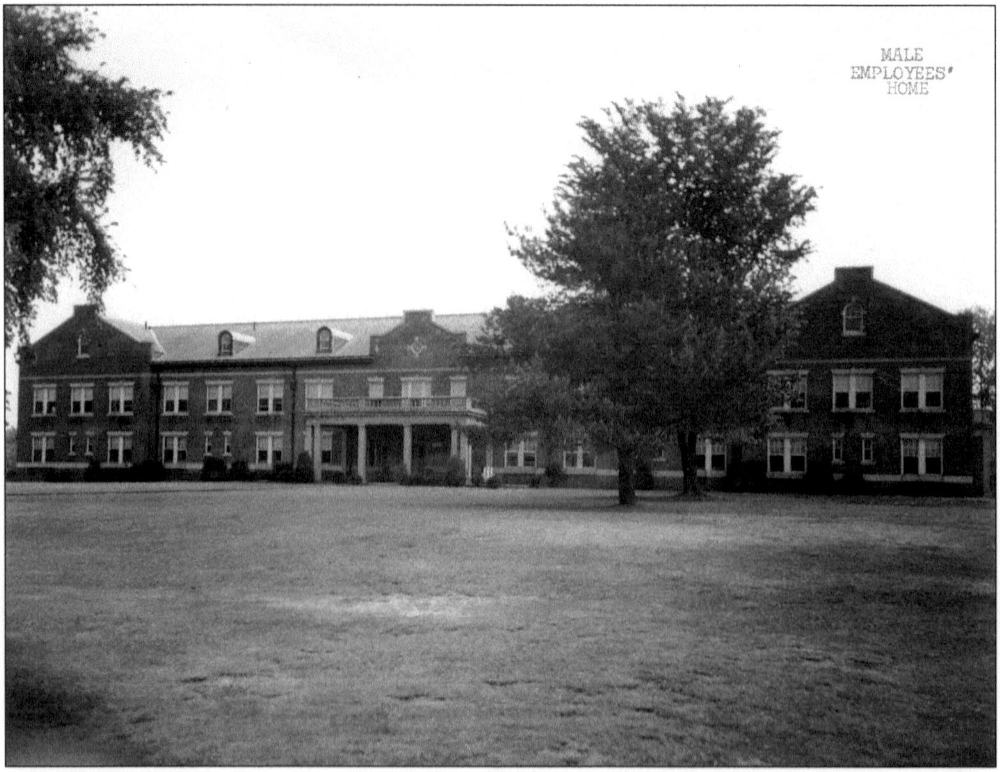

The completed male employees' home is shown above around 1950. Adjacent to it sat the female employees' home, pictured below in 1931. These two buildings, in addition to more on-campus housing for nurses and physicians, sat across from the main hospital campus along Route 12. The male and female employees' homes were nearly identical in exterior construction. (Above, courtesy of Brian Girasoli; below, courtesy of Preston Historical Society.)

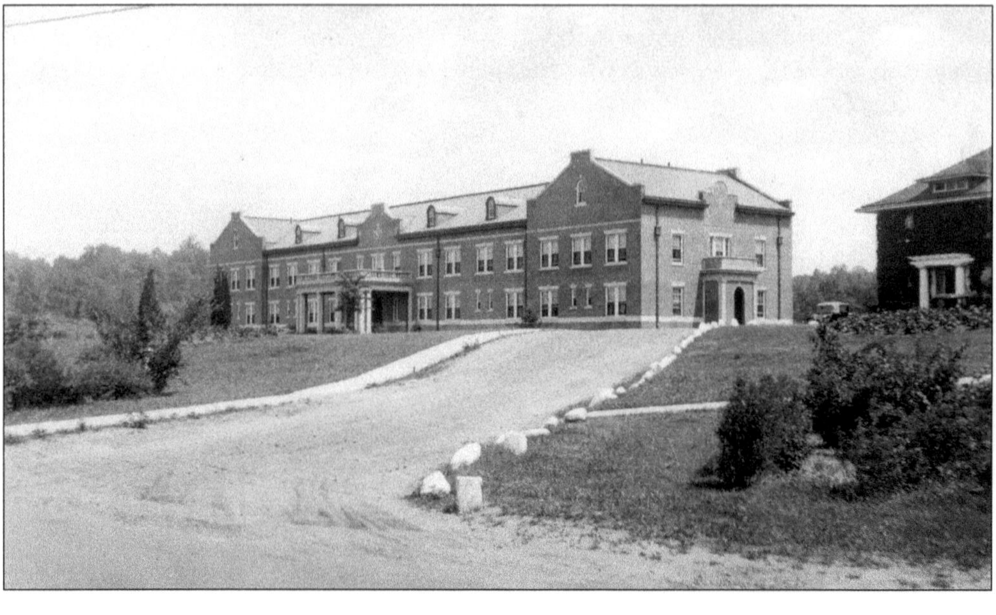

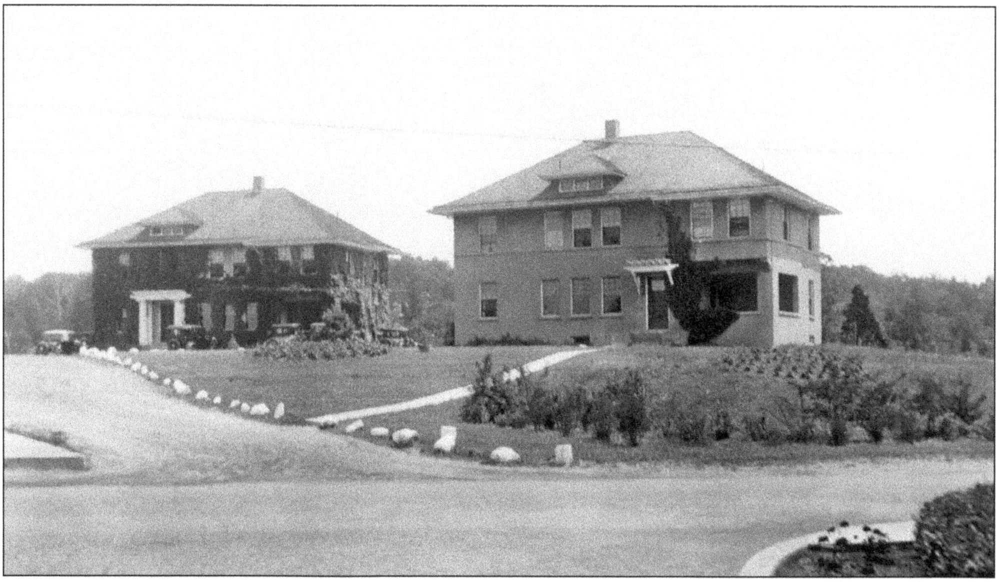

The two nurses' cottages shown above in 1931 were erected in 1910. They sat adjacent to the female employees' home. As the hospital census continued to steadily climb, a third nurses' home, pictured below around 1950, was added to the on-campus employee housing complex by 1939. More patients meant the need for more staff. Work as an attendant in a mental hospital was not seen as an optimal career choice during this period, so like other state hospitals throughout the country, Norwich State Hospital offered attractive on-campus housing for a low weekly rate. (Above, courtesy of Preston Historical Society; below, courtesy of Lloyd Langhammer.)

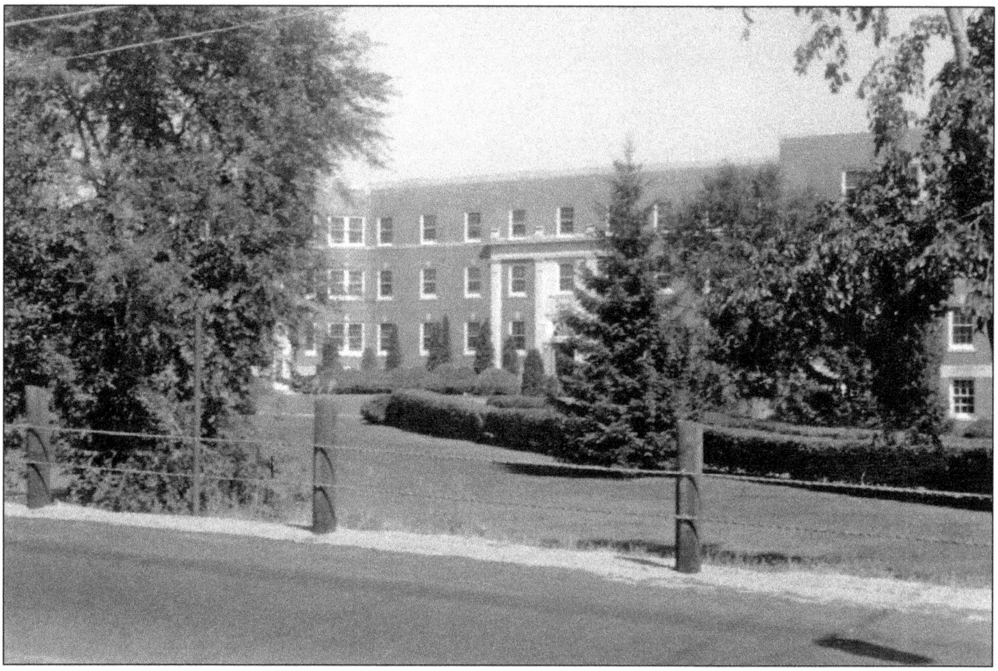

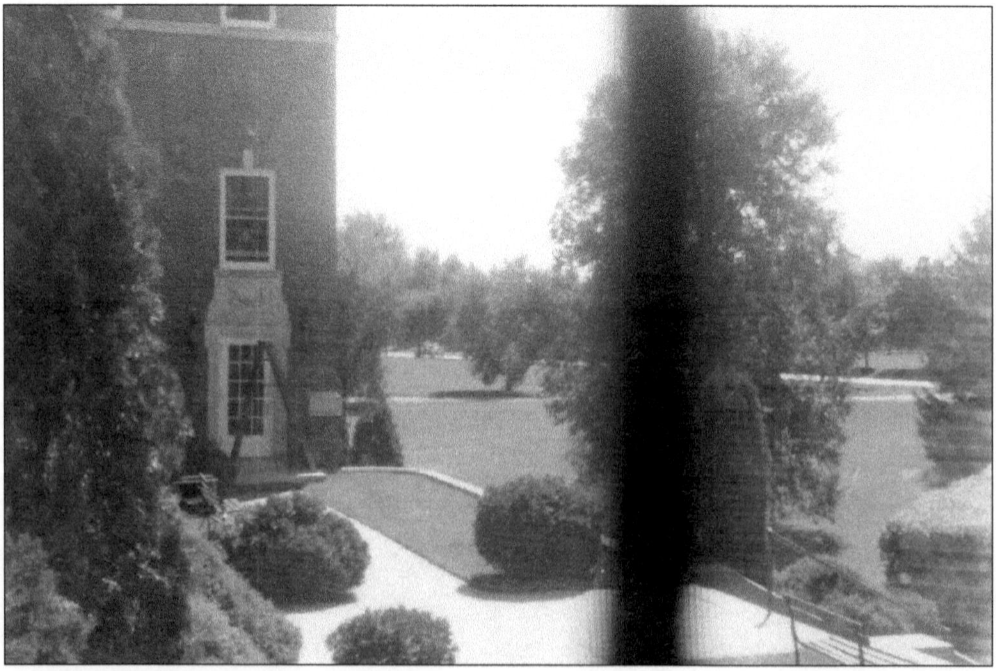

The view above from inside the nurse's home shows a small portion of the well-manicured grounds Norwich State Hospital was highly noted for throughout the surrounding community. Teams of hospital staff and patients took great care in the hospital's physical appearance and in the vegetable and flower gardens shown outside the Lippitt Building below. The food grown in the gardens was used in the hospital's kitchens to prepare meals, and flowers grown in the greenhouse and outdoor beds were used to beautify the wards. (Above, courtesy of Lloyd Langhammer; below, courtesy of Preston Historical Society.)

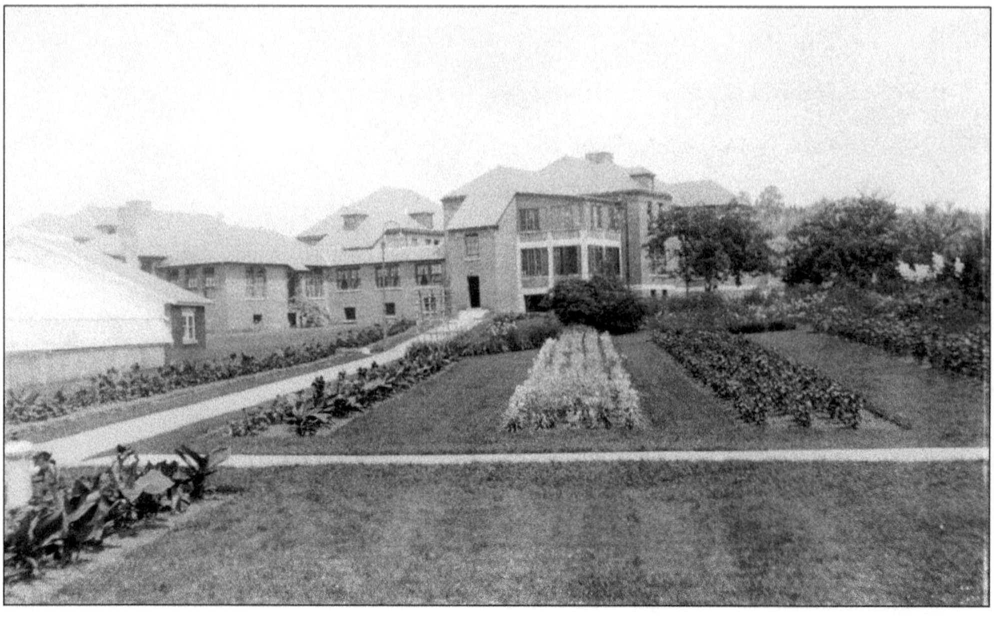

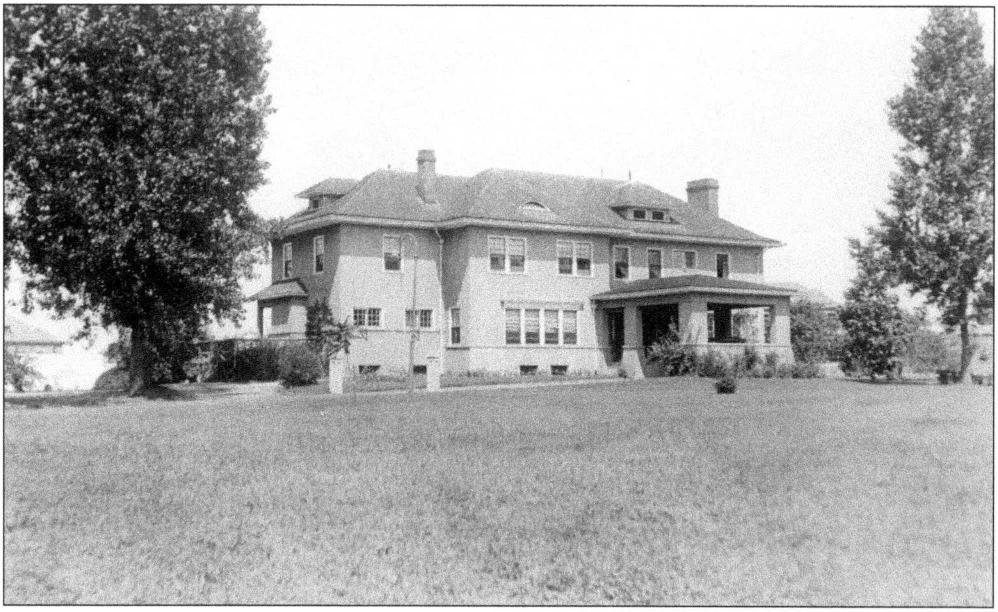

A lavish home for the hospital superintendent and his family sat on the northern side of the main hospital grounds, pictured above in 1931. The assistant superintendent and his family occupied a home similar in size and appearance toward the southern end of the grounds. Shown below is one of the many physicians' cottages that dotted the area surrounding the Lippitt Building. (Both, courtesy of Preston Historical Society.)

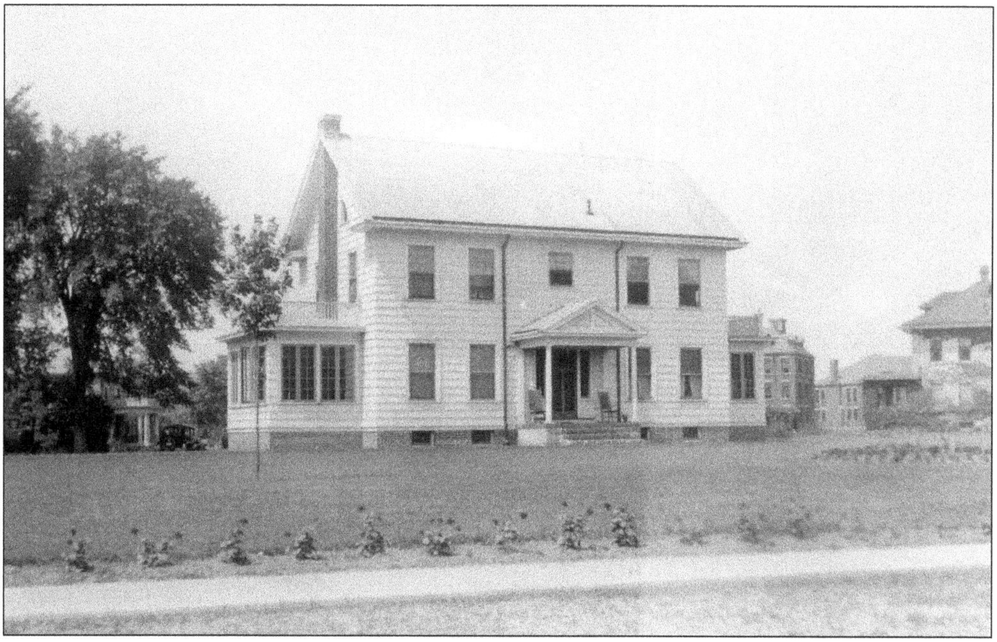

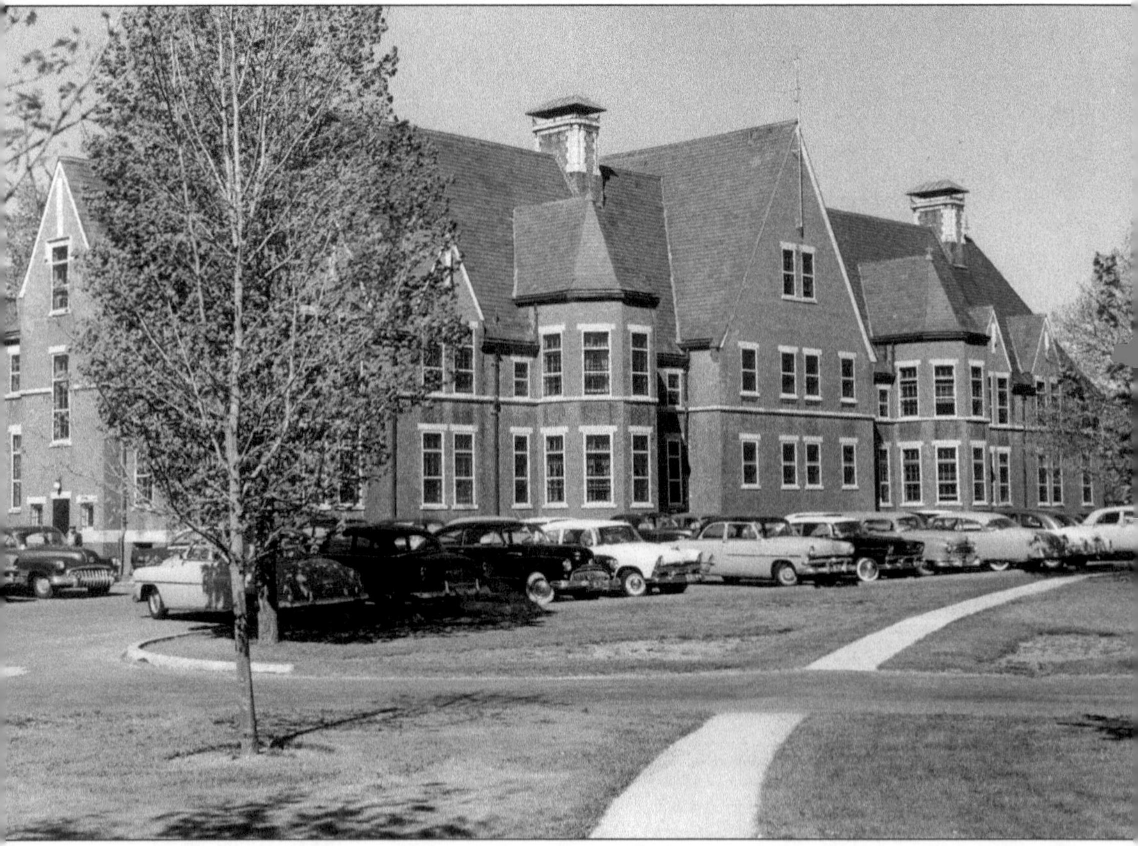

Prior to the establishment of Norwich State Hospital, the state did not have an appropriate place to house criminally insane patients. They were held in regular jails, which were not equipped for handling this type of patient. Since the hospital's opening, each superintendent continuously appealed against the General Assembly's consistent desire to house a criminally insane facility on Norwich State Hospital grounds. The superintendents felt that a special facility needed to be created elsewhere for the therapeutic benefit of this class of patient. The General Assembly eventually won this argument, and in 1937, the second floor of Ward A South was renovated with barred iron doors on each cell and iron fencing separating the wards to house the state's criminally insane. The first floor was given over to forensic research. Ward A South can be seen here retrofitted with iron bars on its windows during the 1950s. (Courtesy of Brian Girasoli.)

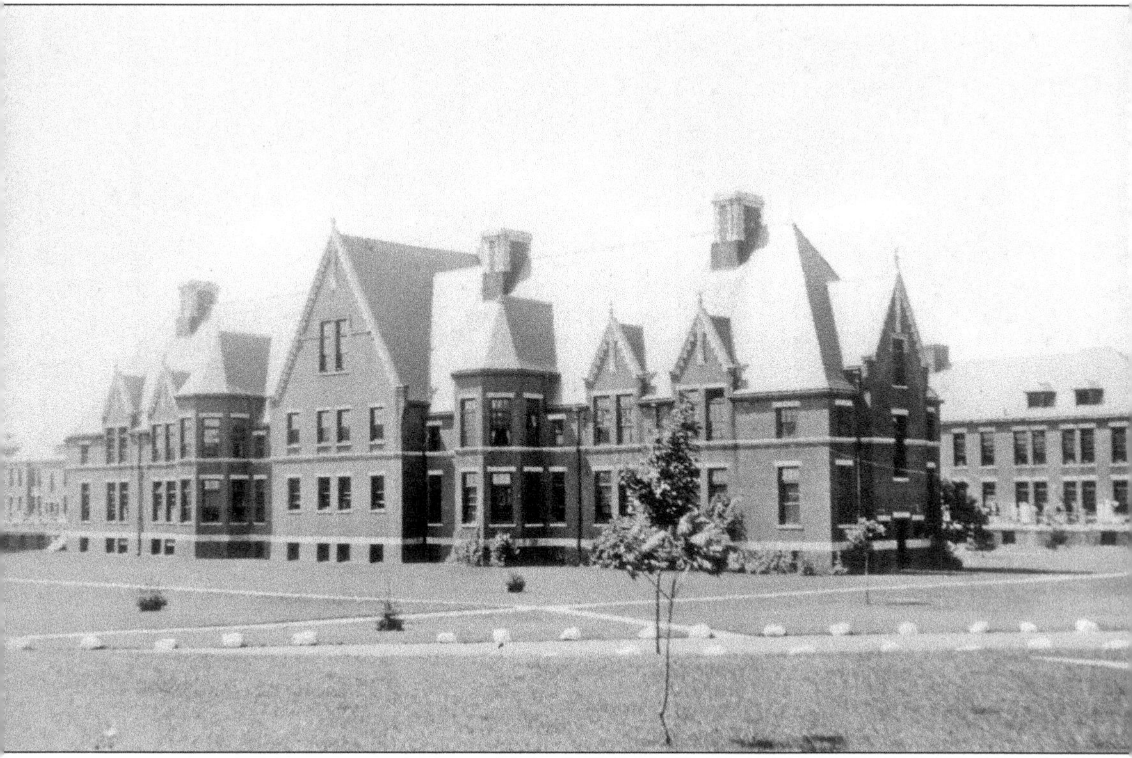

Ward A North is seen here in 1931. It was known as the "Parlor Ward" because the female patients of this building were permitted to have bureaus and personal items, unlike patients on the other wards. This was the only ward where women had any degree of privacy. The patients here had grounds privileges and were good workers. Patients of this class today would never see the inside of a psychiatric institution and would receive any necessary therapeutic treatment on an outpatient basis. The second floor housed attendants and employees who worked in the laundry building and dining rooms. (Courtesy of Preston Historical Society.)

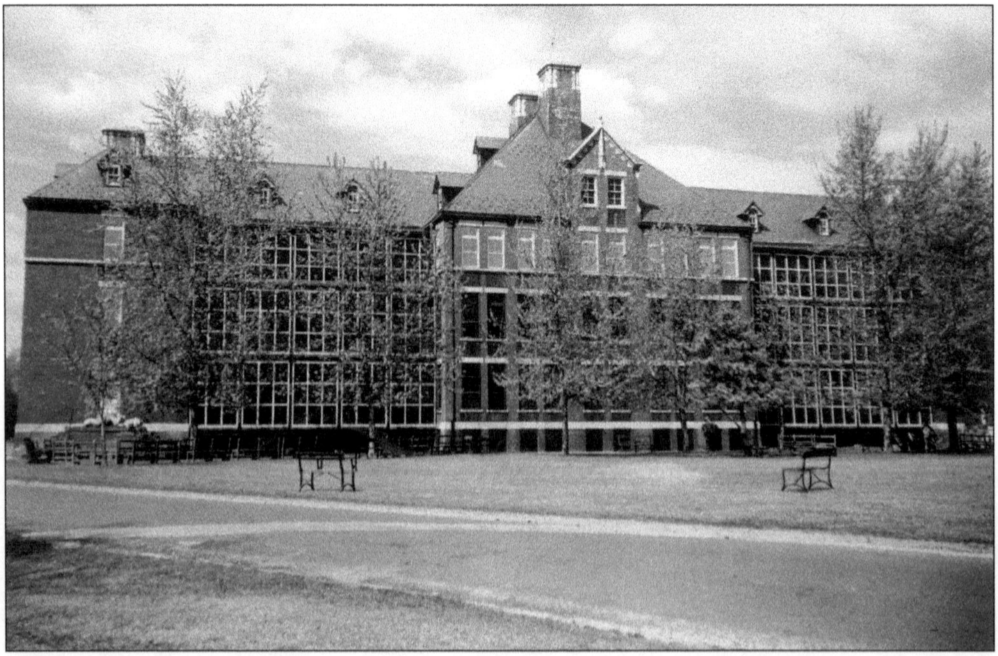

Ward B North (seen above in the 1950s) and Ward B South (below, in 1931) housed 300 chronically ill patients each. Some of these patients had grounds privileges. Noisier patients spent their days on the enclosed grilled porches. These patients were seen as "entertainment" for the public who often toured the grounds on Sundays. (Above, courtesy of Brian Girasoli; below, courtesy of Preston Historical Society.)

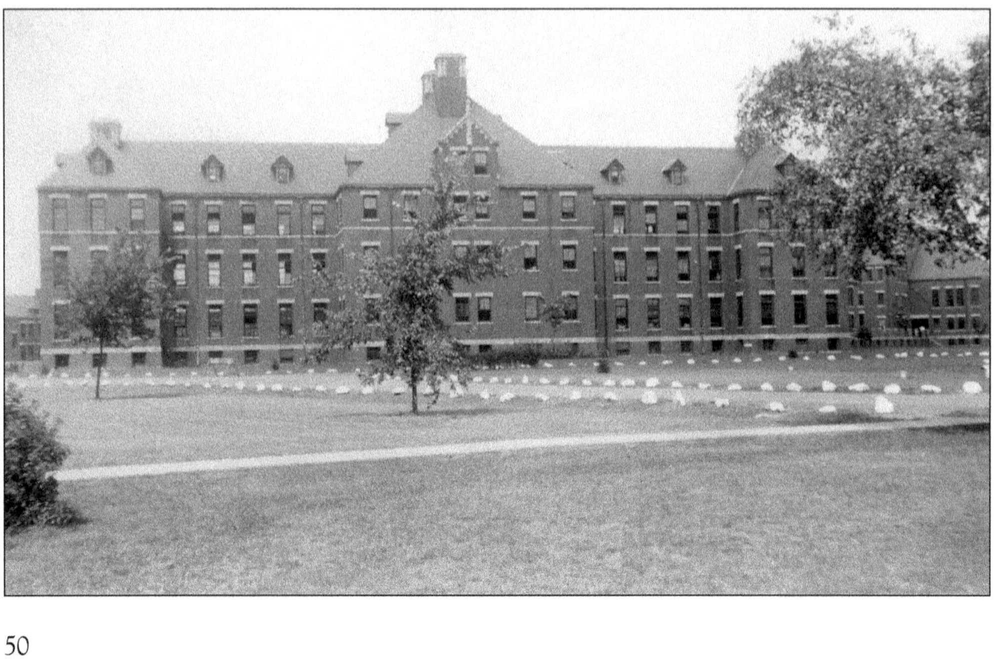

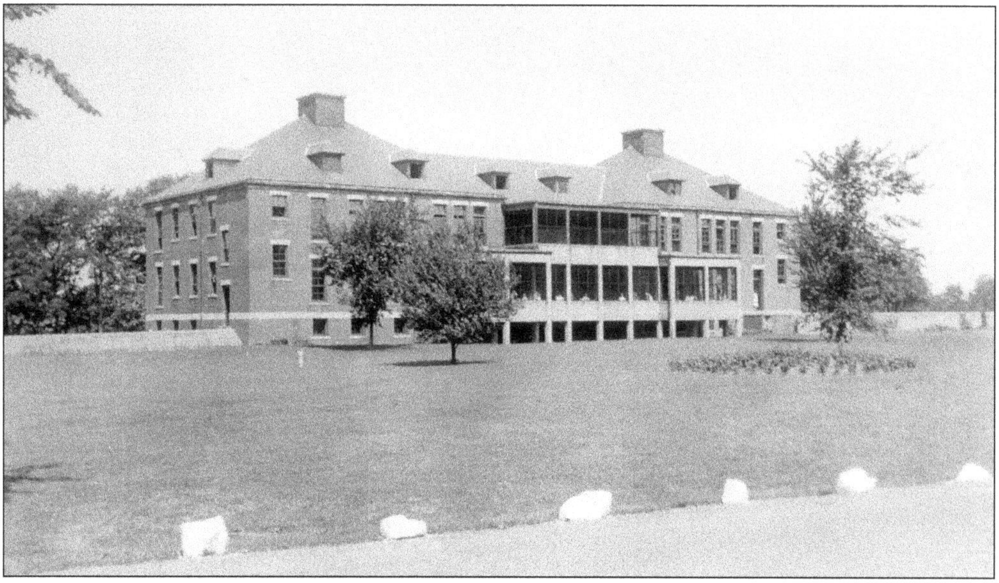

Wards C North (above) and South (below) housed semi-violent female and male patients, respectively. The buildings were poorly furnished, poorly kept, and overcrowded. In the winter, patients who acted out were kept on the cold porches with the doors locked. They could be heard shouting and screaming obscenities. Conditions on Ward C South were inhumane and notoriously the worst in the hospital. Benches were arranged in a circle and patients were ordered never to leave this circle for any reason except meals. Patients who could not control their eliminative functions soiled themselves where they stood. They were sent to the second floor if they tore their clothes, and no new clean clothing was given to them. Beds jammed in together claimed every inch of space on the wards, leaving little to no room to move around. (Above, courtesy of Preston Historical Society; below, courtesy of Brian Girasoli.)

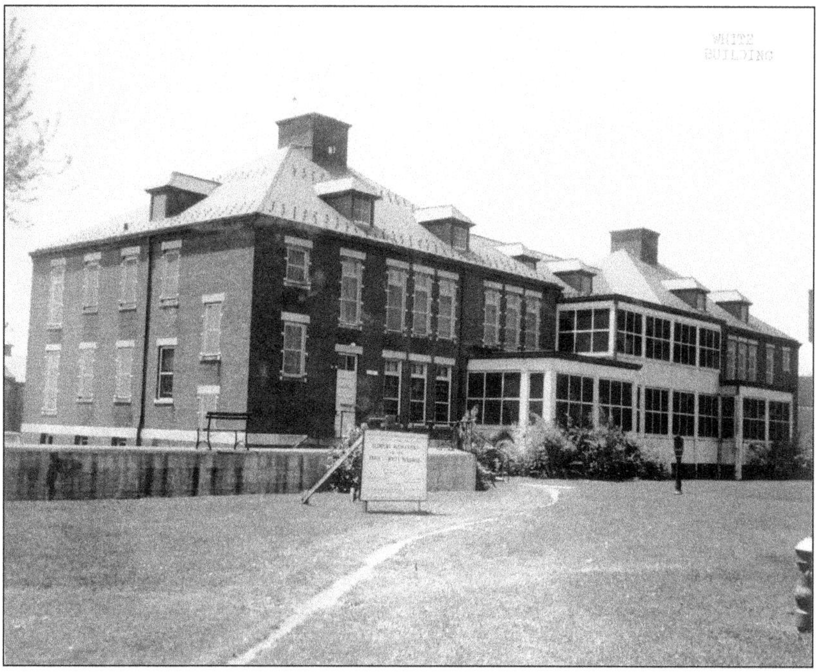

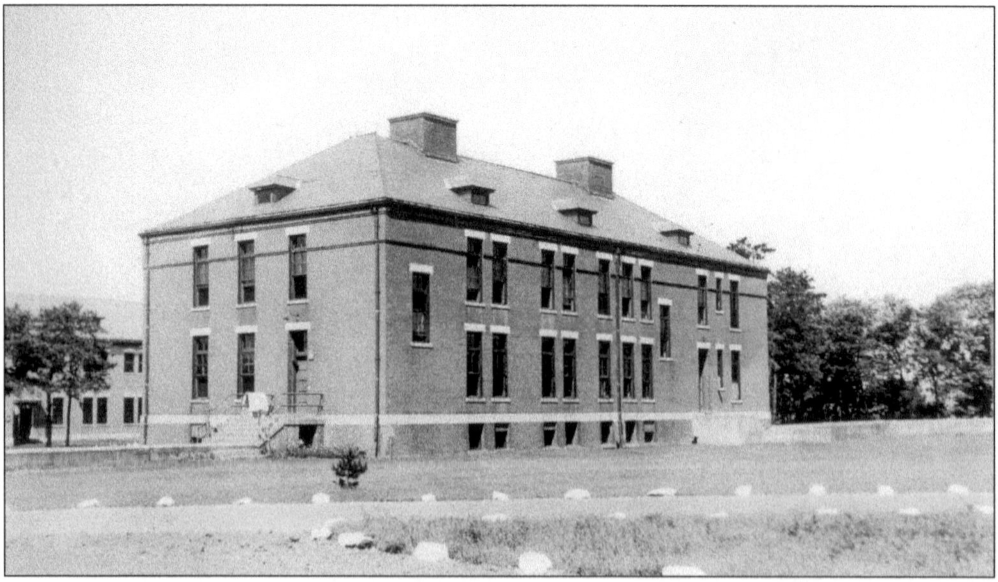

Wards D North (above) and South (below) were the hospital's "violent wards." Overcrowded conditions prevailed here too. Behavior was controlled by sedative medications, wet sheet packs, restraints, and seclusion. Patients in either building could be found tied to benches, asleep on the floors, or standing in a corner without any clothing on. As with Wards C, no partitions were offered between the stalls in the buildings' toilet facilities. (Both, courtesy of Preston Historical Society.)

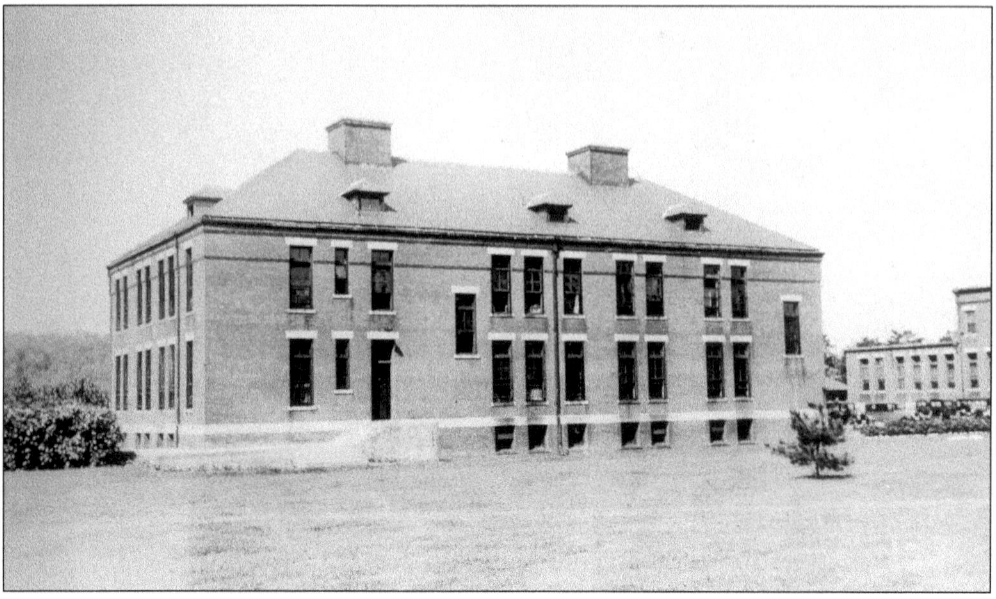

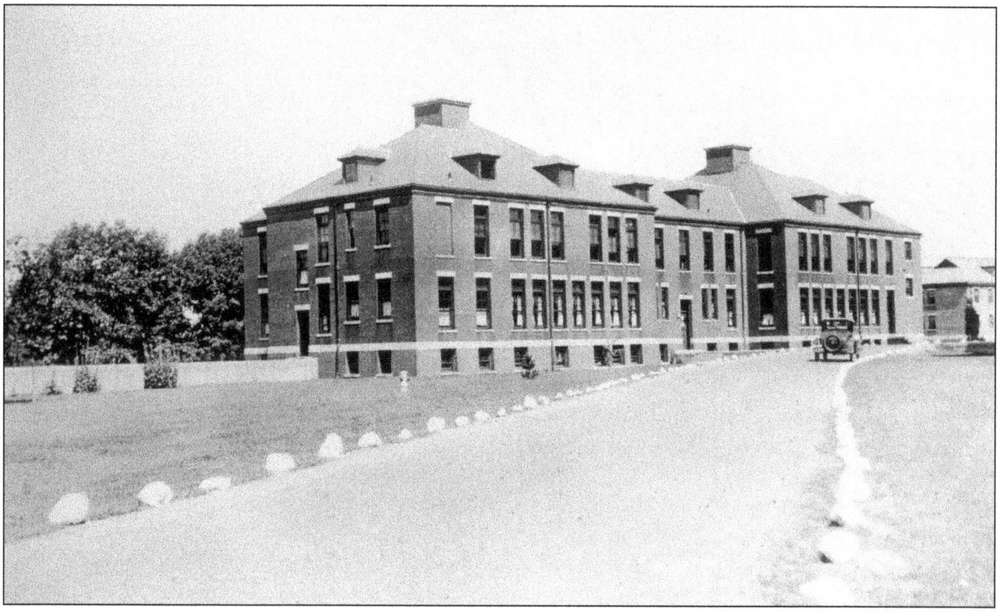

Wards E North (above) and South (below) housed epileptic patients. Both buildings were in excess of their 100 patient capacities. Patients who had frequent severe seizures were tied to a bench during the day in an attempt to prevent injuries that might be sustained during a seizure. Patients here were dressed in "strong dresses," camisoles, or unattractive, ill-fitting state clothing. Those who lashed out were placed in seclusion. In 1931, there were no medications to control the seizures except for bromides and phenobarbital, and neither was very effective. (Both, courtesy of Preston Historical Society.)

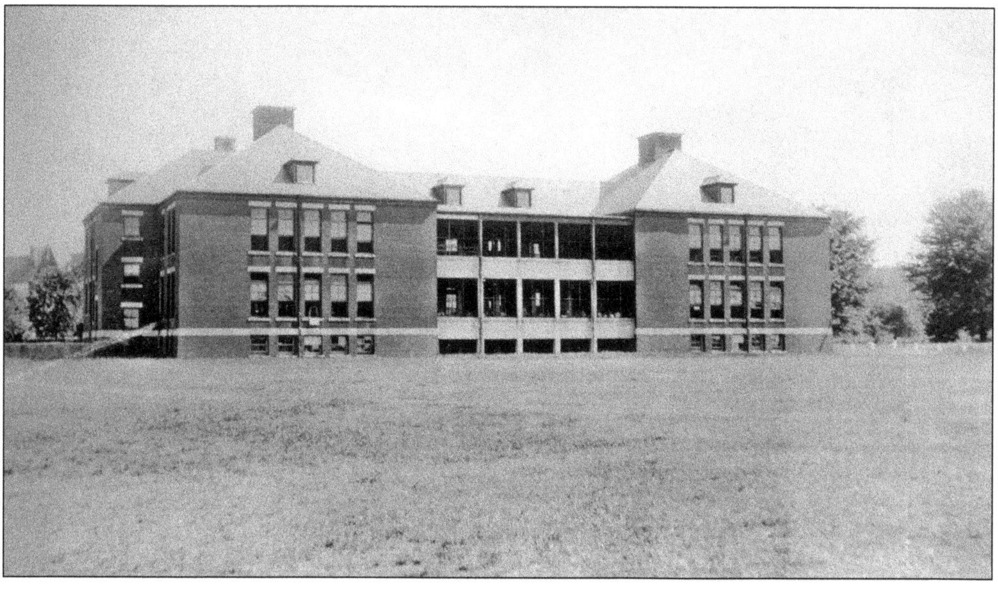

Insofar as the report of the "Commission on the Treatment and Care of People Afflicted with Physical or Mental Disabilities" concerns itself with the charge made in the State Senate May 31, 1939, that the Norwich State Hospital "stinks to high heaven", it demon-

The aforementioned conditions were some of the reasons why Sen. Joseph B. Downes charged that the Norwich State Hospital "stinks to high heaven" in the state senate on May 31, 1939. As neat as the dormitory shown in 1930 appears below, little to no room was provided for movement and comfort between each bed. Dorms such as these would become home to nearly twice as many beds as the 1930s wore on, worsening the poor living conditions Downes complained of. Additional accusations of patient mistreatment and staff mismanagement prompted the Public Welfare Council to form the Commission on the Treatment and Care of People Afflicted with Physical or Mental Disabilities, also known as the Barker Commission. It conducted lengthy investigations into the hospital to support Downes's allegations. Superintendent Waterman launched his own investigation to counter the accusations. A snippet from Superintendent Waterman's independent investigation from 1939 is pictured above. The Barker Commission's investigation lasted four months. (Above, author's collection; below, courtesy of Connecticut State Library.)

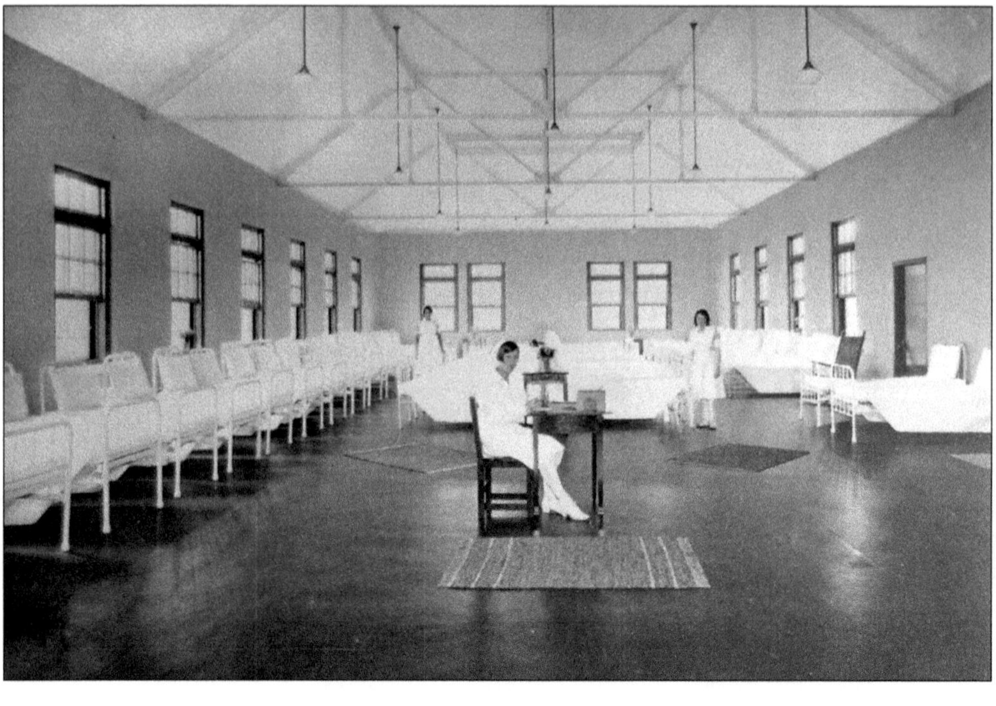

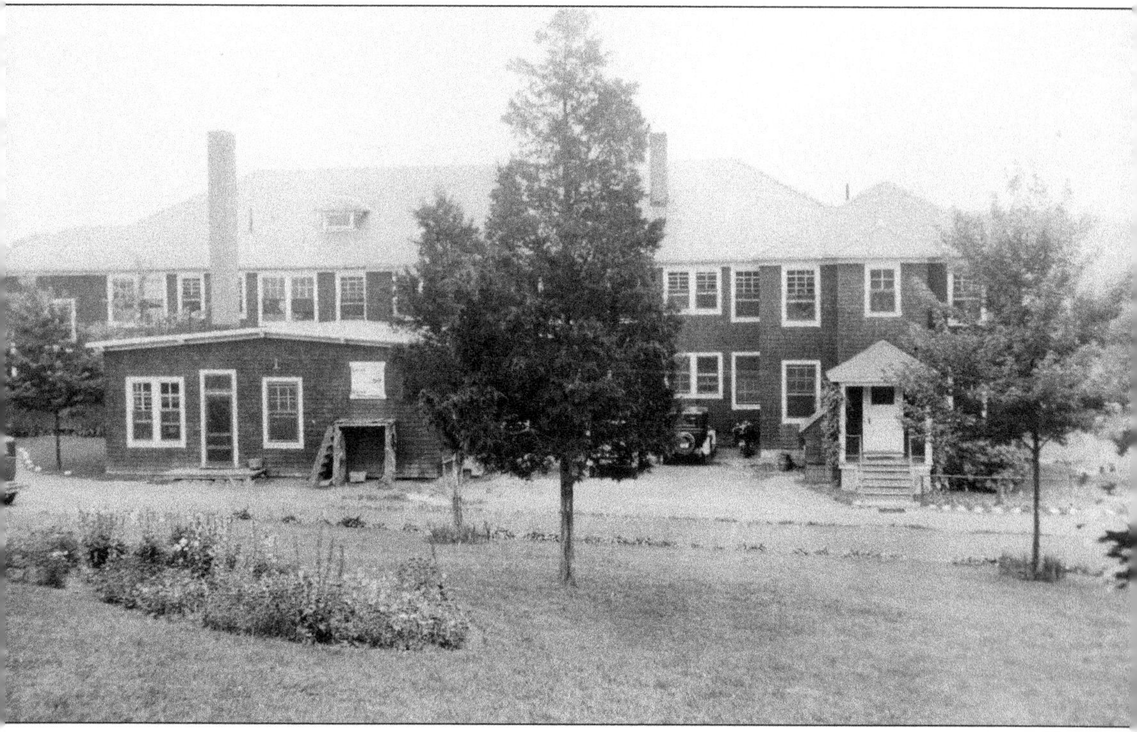

One of the findings in the Barker Commission's report was that the tuberculosis building, known as "The Pines," was grossly neglected and a fire hazard. Conditions and management inside were found to be worse. The 100 patients housed here were under the care of only one physician, who had two other wards in his charge. This physician had no education or training in treating tubercular cases, and he rarely visited the ward. Little consultation was made with the nearby Uncas on Thames tuberculosis hospital to help the patients. Hospital records showed that the clinical director had not visited The Pines more than four to five times in the past four to five years. (Courtesy of Preston Historical Society.)

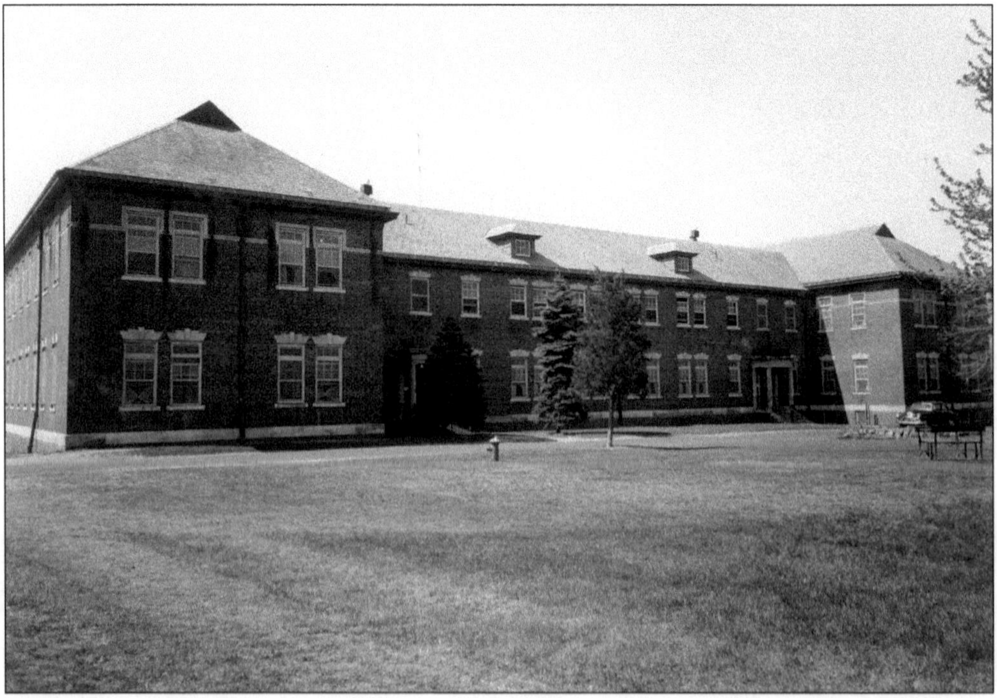

Ward South K (above) and Ward North H (below) were infirmaries for senile men and women, respectively. The pungent odor of urine and disinfectants filled each building. Beds were tightly jammed together against the walls. The patients of these wards lay in their beds frail, depressed, and waiting for death. The conditions on these wards also helped to support the allegations made by the Barker Commission. (Above, courtesy of Brian Girasoli; below, courtesy of Preston Historical Society.)

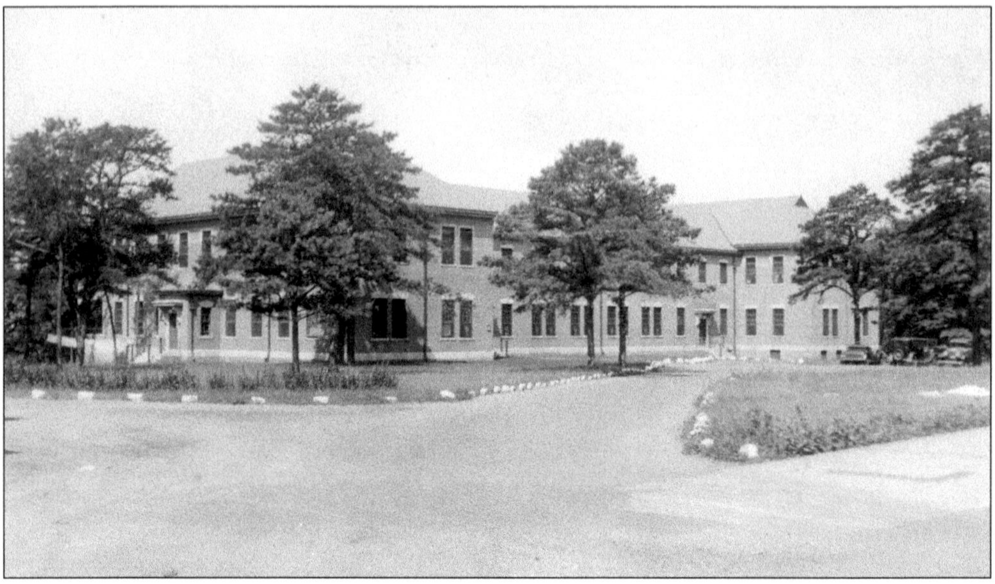

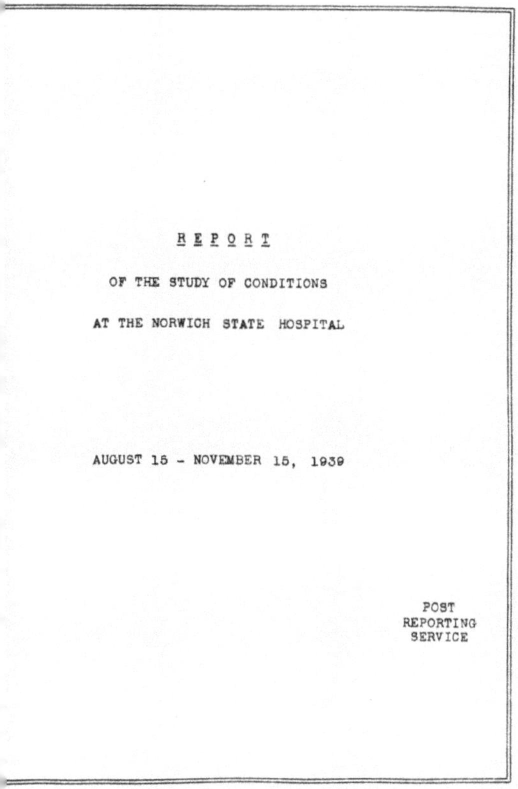

REPORT

OF THE STUDY OF CONDITIONS

AT THE NORWICH STATE HOSPITAL

AUGUST 15 - NOVEMBER 15, 1939

POST
REPORTING
SERVICE

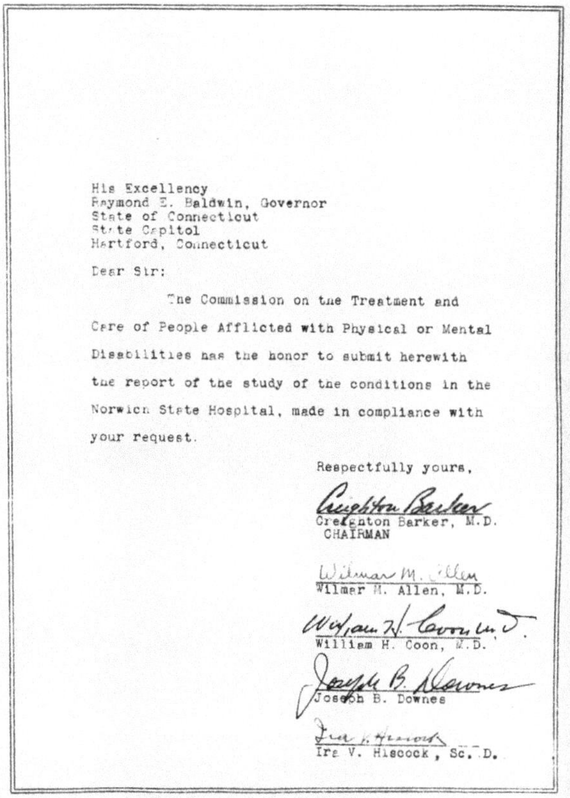

His Excellency
Raymond E. Baldwin, Governor
State of Connecticut
State Capitol
Hartford, Connecticut

Dear Sir:

The Commission on the Treatment and Care of People Afflicted with Physical or Mental Disabilities has the honor to submit herewith the report of the study of the conditions in the Norwich State Hospital, made in compliance with your request.

Respectfully yours,

Creighton Barker, M.D.
CHAIRMAN

Wilmar M. Allen, M.D.

William H. Coon, M.D.

Joseph B. Downes

Ira V. Hiscock, Sc. D.

The Barker Commission's report to the governor of Connecticut found the hospital to be severely mismanaged and that it did not meet the minimum requirements for accreditation with the American Psychiatric Association. The report further stated that a frequent comment made by employees around the hospital was that "the business manager runs the hospital." The business manager was indeed found to have more administrative power than the superintendent. Ward employees were strategically parking their personal cars in back of ward buildings and were using them to steal supplies that were desperately needed on the wards. The medical staff was found to be inadequate both in quality and quantity. Diagnostic lab procedures were not being completed. During interviews, both the superintendent and clinical director admitted that some of the medical staff members were known to be incompetent and that their work was unsatisfactory, but no effort was made to correct this. The assistant superintendent "expressed himself as never having been quite sure of what his duties were." Patients were found to be insufficiently clothed and not properly nourished, and physical abuses of them were found to be infrequent and promptly and strictly dealt with. (Author's collection.)

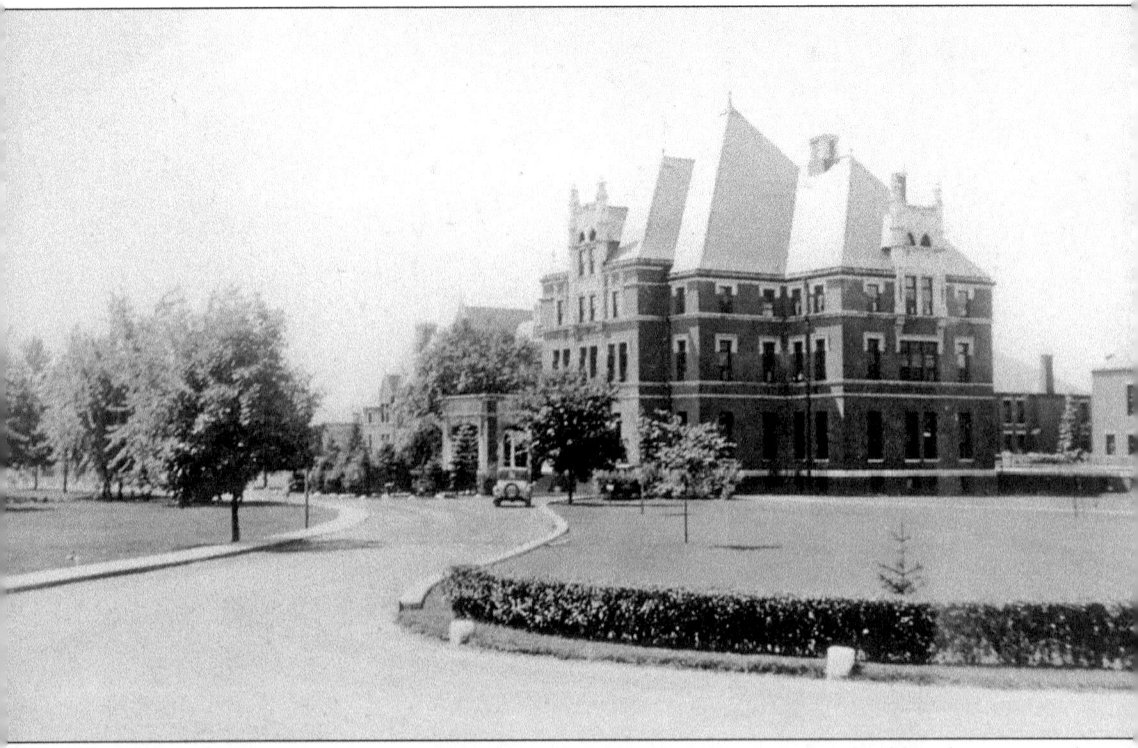

Ward physicians were discovered to have offices in the Administration Building but not on the wards in their charge. Ward reports and hospital records were not being kept. There was much hostility among the medical staff due to the lack of a strong superintendent leader. The Barker Commission and Dr. Waterman's own investigative committee made several recommendations for improvement of the hospital and its administration. Dr. Waterman agreed with some of the recommendations and disagreed with others. Dr. Waterman submitted his resignation in the face of the commission's investigations. His resignation was accepted by the board of trustees and made effective May 1, 1940. (Courtesy of Preston Historical Society.)

Three

Hospital Changes and World War II

Dr. William A. Bryan was selected to head NSH by the board of trustees following Dr. Waterman's resignation during the Barker Commission's investigation. As the investigations neared a close, the Public Welfare Council issued a public statement on December 8, 1939, that Dr. Waterman and the board of trustees should not be blamed for conditions at the hospital. The council charged that the fault lay with the General Assembly for failing to provide sufficient appropriations, which forced the hospital into unfair economizing. Dr. Waterman neglected to state a reason for his resignation but publicly stated "I have nothing to apologize for. I have done my duty as my training and experience of 35 years gave me the ability to do. I take justifiable pride in leaving the institution a vastly better place for the health and happiness of patients than it was when I came to the hospital."

Dr. Bryan was a dynamic and energetic man who brought a tidal wave of positive energy to Norwich State Hospital. He immediately instituted massive change throughout the whole hospital and set high standards for all employees to follow. He reclassified every patient ward and reorganized every hospital department. New systems for detailed, accurate record keeping were implemented. He frequently made rounds and visited the wards day and night. He had no tolerance for employees who neglected patients and was known to dismiss them on the spot. He demanded patients no longer be kept solely indoors and had chairs and benches placed outside on the grounds for them to use at will. Staff resisted this new change, but Dr. Bryan personally intervened and ensured that patients be able to move about the grounds freely without constricting supervision. He courageously led the hospital through the hardships of World War II. Even in his physical absence, his presence could be felt at every level.

Dr. Bryan would only superintend Norwich State Hospital for four years before his death in 1944, but in that short time, he exerted a great influence on the hospital's future growth and development.

Return Postage Guaranteed, Box 508, Norwich, Conn. Sec. 562, P. L. & R.

THE STYLUS

OF

THE NORWICH STATE HOSPITAL. NORWICH, CONN.

Vol. 2 MARCH 1, 1942 No. 3

ESCAPES

Two elements make a modern progressive mental hospital. First, a hospital staff that is sincere, energetic and filled with determination to find a better treatment than that used yesterday. Second, a community that will loyally support the hospital and be receptive to education in the importance of changing treatment procedures.

The problem of escapes from mental hospitals illustrates the importance of these two elements. It would be entirely possible for any hospital staff to organize its institution like a prison so that escapes were rare or impossible. In fact, such an organization would make the work and responsibilities of the staff far easier. It so happens, however, that such treatment is not only inhumane, but does not promote recovery from mental illness.

The community attitude is just as important as that of the hospital staff. Many citizens read with horror the news that a patient has escaped. Those who know the facts realize there is no reason to be afraid. The number of patients who escape is low in proportion to the large and increasing number of patients enjoying freedom of the grounds. During the last six months patients enjoying this freedom increased about 60%, whereas during the same period the percentage of escapes showed no important change.

Is there danger to the community in these escapes? Actually, to our knowledge, no escaped patient has injured anyone at all during the past five years. Let us realize too, that the average number of escapes from the hospital per month is only one out of 400 patients.

A sensible approach to understanding the significance of these escaped patients is to ask what these

Continued on Page 2, Column 3

Monthly Memo

Quite frequently, of late, I have been asked if the war and social conditions caused by it are causing an increase in the amount of mental illness. The best answer I can give is that there is no evidence of an increase.

We can be fairly certain that the increase in employment, with full dinner pails for more people, has saved many people from breaking under strains produced by poverty and untreated physical illness.

However, we should say, also, that any social readjustments required by war-time conditions put an unusual strain of anxiety and worry, resulting in mental breakdown in many people who would otherwise be able to get along without psychiatric help.

Many of us have a tendency to evade the unpleasant realities of life. What we need is to face realities, calmly and fearlessly, to accept responsibilities, to understand the world as it is and to do something about the unpleasant things. Thus we keep our balance and even increase our mental and emotional strength.

WILLIAM A. BRYAN, M. D.,
Superintendent.

"Service Buttons" for March

Emil Bausch—28 years.
Anna E. Burdick—27 years.
Frederick W. Kindall—19 years.
Anthony Wesloski—19 years.
Ethel Smith—17 years.
Joseph F. Smith—17 years.
George Mansfield—16 years.
Charles Olin—15 years.
William S. Parker—14 years.
James W. Southouse—14 years.
Anthony Masalsky—11 years.
Helen B. Nawrocky—11 years.
William Partridge—11 years.

American Medical Association Approves Norwich State Hospital

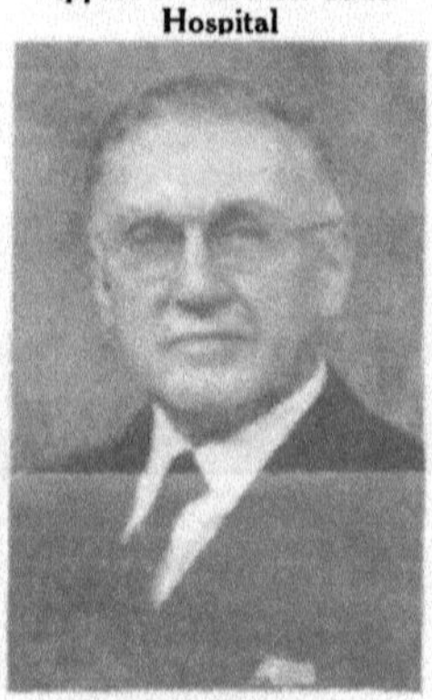

DR. WILLIAM A. BRYAN
Superintendant

The Council of the American Medical Association at its meeting in Chicago, February 15th, certified the Norwich State Hospital as an educational center for resident training of doctors in psychiatry. This approval was dated as of May first, 1941, which was exactly one year after Dr. Bryan took the post as Superintendent, and is a distinctive recognition of his intensive efforts to make this one of the outstanding mental hospitals of the nation.

This recognition means not only that Norwich State Hospital is highly accredited for its scientific care and treatment of mental illness, but also, that doctors may come here for training and experience to qualify as Diplomates of the American Board of Psychiatry and Neurology.

As the basis for this certification, The American Medical Association

Continued on Page 4. Column 2

Dr. William A. Bryan led Norwich State Hospital from 1940 until his death in 1944. His portrait is seen here in the ninth issue of the hospital's first self-published newsletter, *The Stylus*. Dr. Bryan was highly educated and brought a wealth of psychiatric hospital experience to Norwich State Hospital. He began his career as an attendant at state hospitals in Iowa. He proudly shared his early career experiences with his Norwich State Hospital staff, urging them not to cut corners because he "knew all the ropes." He was very selective with hiring new staff and took great care to weed out the "hospital tramps," people who were known to move from one state hospital job to another after being disciplined or terminated for patient neglect and abuse. He was briefly assistant superintendent at Danvers State Hospital in Massachusetts before becoming superintendent of Worcester State Hospital. Dr. Bryan was highly esteemed for his revolutionary work over 20 years at Worcester before coming to Norwich State Hospital. (Courtesy of Connecticut State Library.)

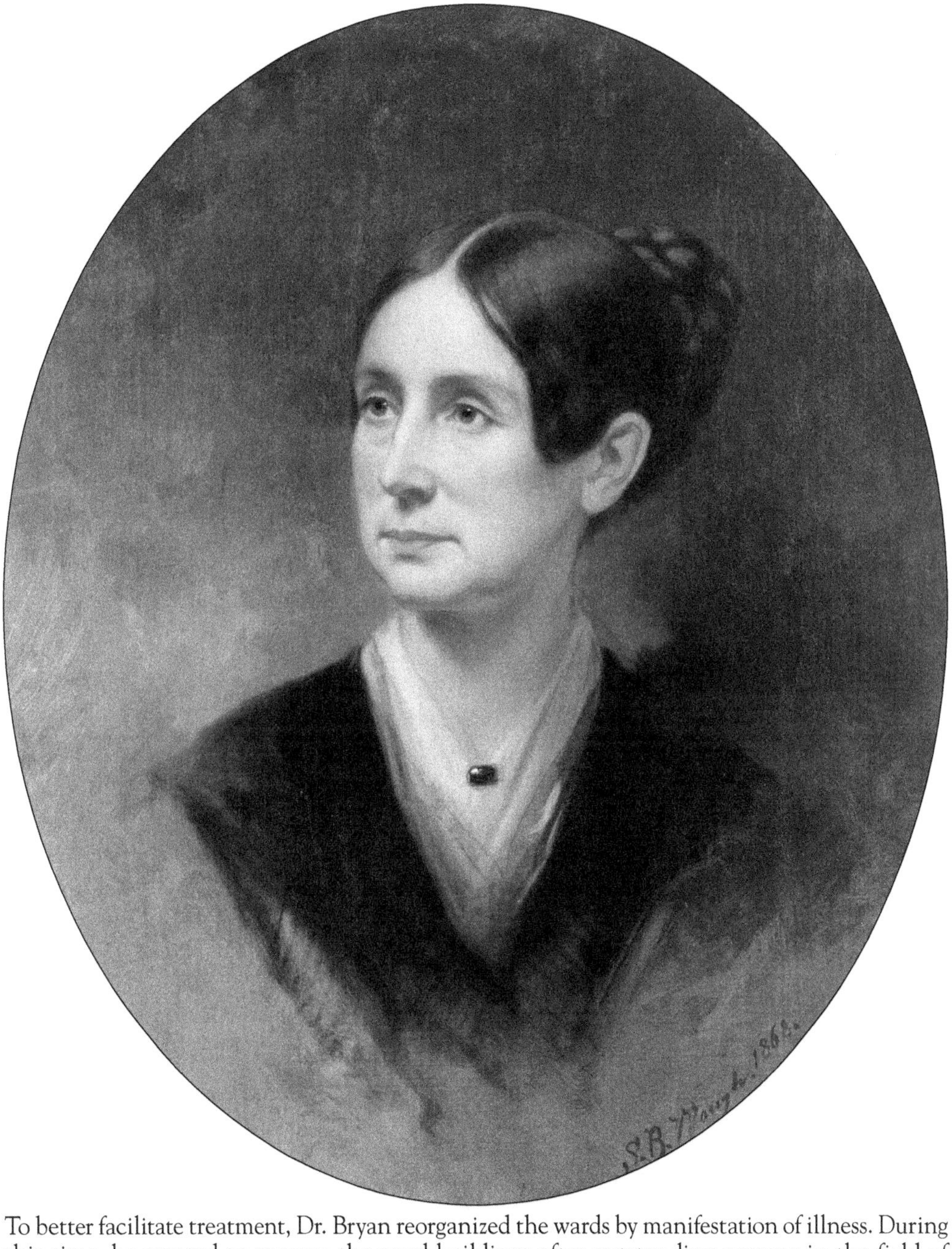

To better facilitate treatment, Dr. Bryan reorganized the wards by manifestation of illness. During this time, he wanted to rename the ward buildings after outstanding persons in the field of psychiatry. The board of trustees gave its approval for the change with the stipulation that the buildings that had already been named—Gallup, Lippitt, and Seymour—were not to be changed. Pictured here is Dorothea Dix, an American activist who lobbied state legislatures on behalf of indigent mentally ill persons for better care and treatment in state hospitals. She also aided in the creation of the first generation of psychiatric hospitals. With the renaming of the buildings, Ward D North became the Dix Building. (Author's collection.)

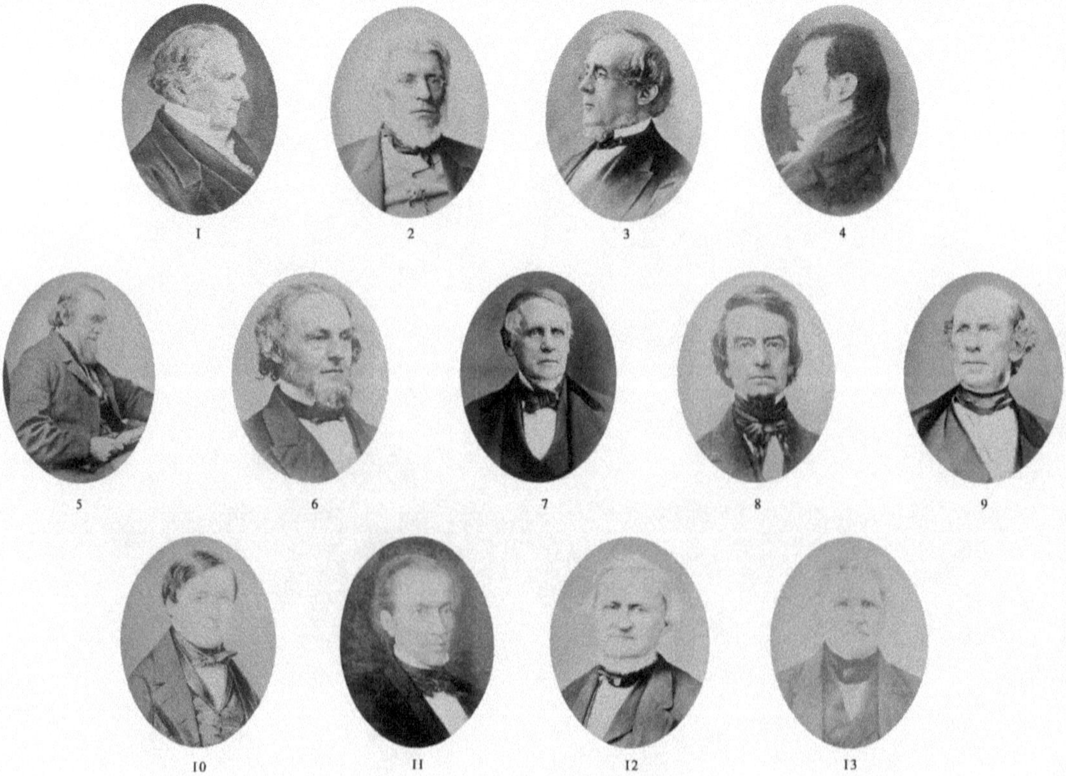

THE ORIGINAL THIRTEEN

(1) Samuel B. Woodward, (2) Isaac Ray, (3) John S. Butler, (4) Samuel White, (5) Charles H. Stedman, (6) Pliny Earle, (7) Thomas S. Kirkbride, (8) Luther V. Bell, (9) William L. Awl, (10), John M. Galt, (11) Amariah Brigham, (12) Francis T. Stribling, (13) Nehemiah Cutter.

Pictured are the 13 founding members of the Association of Medical Superintendents of American Institutions for the Insane, which is known today as the American Psychiatric Association (APA). The names of the founding members and their new corresponding wards were, from left to right, (top row) Samuel B. Woodward (Ward F North), Isaac Ray (Ward H North), John S. Butler (Ward E North), and Samuel White (Ward C South); (middle row) Charles H. Stedman (Ward F South), Pliny Earle (Ward E South), Thomas S. Kirkbride (Ward K South) and Luther V. Bell (Ward B North), and William L. Awl (Ward A North); (bottom row) John M. Galt (Ward G South), Amariah Brigham (Ward B South), Francis T. Stribling (Ward D South), and Nehemiah Cutter (Ward C North). Two other wards, Ward G North and Ward A South, were named for two more prominent figures in the history of mental health: S. Weir Mitchell and Dr. Thomas W. Salmon, respectively. (Author's collection.)

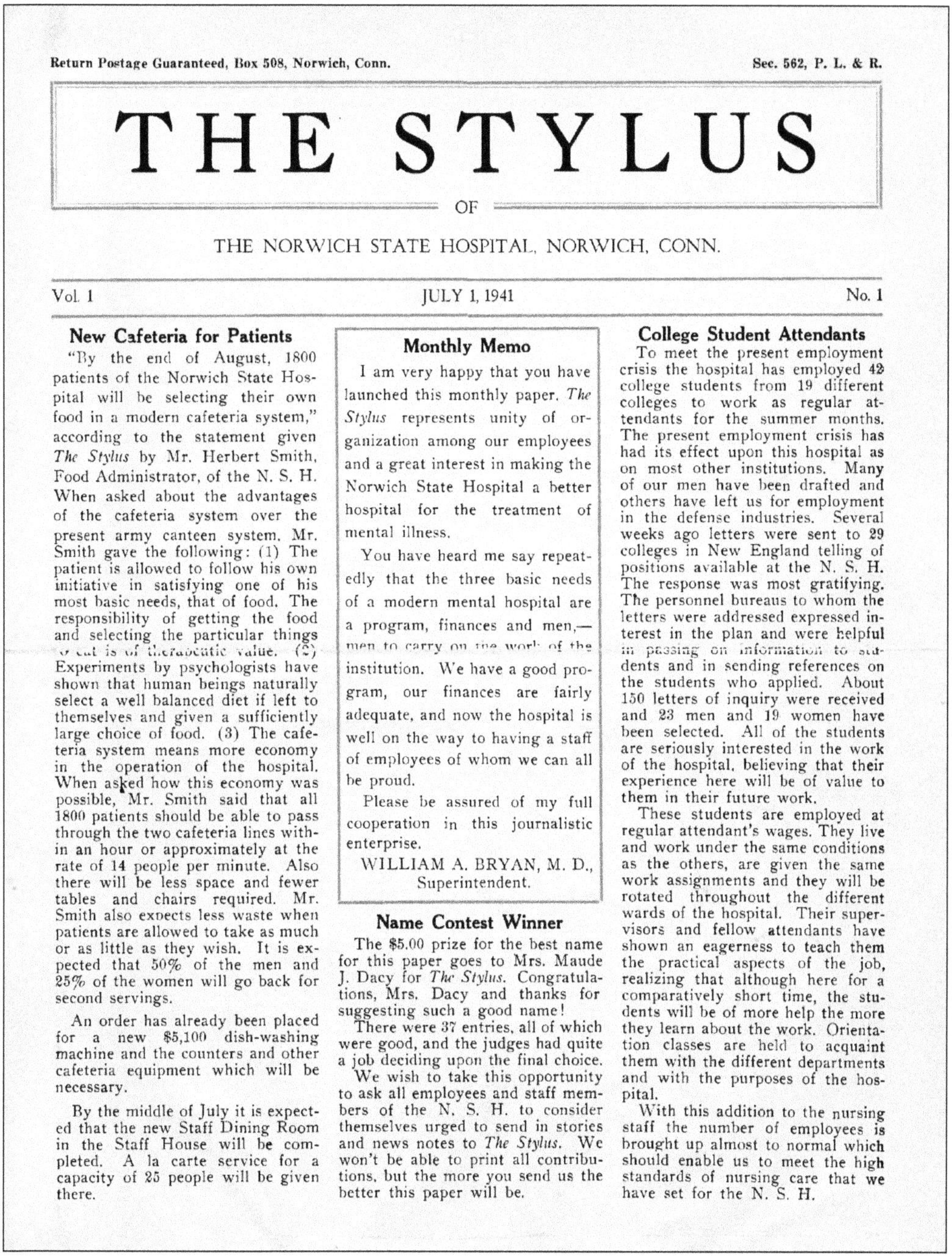

Return Postage Guaranteed, Box 508, Norwich, Conn. Sec. 562, P. L. & R.

THE STYLUS

OF

THE NORWICH STATE HOSPITAL, NORWICH, CONN.

Vol. 1 JULY 1, 1941 No. 1

New Cafeteria for Patients

"By the end of August, 1800 patients of the Norwich State Hospital will be selecting their own food in a modern cafeteria system," according to the statement given *The Stylus* by Mr. Herbert Smith, Food Administrator, of the N. S. H. When asked about the advantages of the cafeteria system over the present army canteen system, Mr. Smith gave the following: (1) The patient is allowed to follow his own initiative in satisfying one of his most basic needs, that of food. The responsibility of getting the food and selecting the particular things that is of therapeutic value. (2) Experiments by psychologists have shown that human beings naturally select a well balanced diet if left to themselves and given a sufficiently large choice of food. (3) The cafeteria system means more economy in the operation of the hospital. When asked how this economy was possible, Mr. Smith said that all 1800 patients should be able to pass through the two cafeteria lines within an hour or approximately at the rate of 14 people per minute. Also there will be less space and fewer tables and chairs required. Mr. Smith also expects less waste when patients are allowed to take as much or as little as they wish. It is expected that 50% of the men and 25% of the women will go back for second servings.

An order has already been placed for a new $5,100 dish-washing machine and the counters and other cafeteria equipment which will be necessary.

By the middle of July it is expected that the new Staff Dining Room in the Staff House will be completed. A la carte service for a capacity of 25 people will be given there.

Monthly Memo

I am very happy that you have launched this monthly paper. *The Stylus* represents unity of organization among our employees and a great interest in making the Norwich State Hospital a better hospital for the treatment of mental illness.

You have heard me say repeatedly that the three basic needs of a modern mental hospital are a program, finances and men,—men to carry on the work of the institution. We have a good program, our finances are fairly adequate, and now the hospital is well on the way to having a staff of employees of whom we can all be proud.

Please be assured of my full cooperation in this journalistic enterprise.

WILLIAM A. BRYAN, M. D.,
Superintendent.

Name Contest Winner

The $5.00 prize for the best name for this paper goes to Mrs. Maude J. Dacy for *The Stylus*. Congratulations, Mrs. Dacy and thanks for suggesting such a good name!

There were 37 entries, all of which were good, and the judges had quite a job deciding upon the final choice.

We wish to take this opportunity to ask all employees and staff members of the N. S. H. to consider themselves urged to send in stories and news notes to *The Stylus*. We won't be able to print all contributions, but the more you send us the better this paper will be.

College Student Attendants

To meet the present employment crisis the hospital has employed 42 college students from 19 different colleges to work as regular attendants for the summer months. The present employment crisis has had its effect upon this hospital as on most other institutions. Many of our men have been drafted and others have left us for employment in the defense industries. Several weeks ago letters were sent to 29 colleges in New England telling of positions available at the N. S. H. The response was most gratifying. The personnel bureaus to whom the letters were addressed expressed interest in the plan and were helpful in passing on information to students and in sending references on the students who applied. About 150 letters of inquiry were received and 23 men and 19 women have been selected. All of the students are seriously interested in the work of the hospital, believing that their experience here will be of value to them in their future work.

These students are employed at regular attendant's wages. They live and work under the same conditions as the others, are given the same work assignments and they will be rotated throughout the different wards of the hospital. Their supervisors and fellow attendants have shown an eagerness to teach them the practical aspects of the job, realizing that although here for a comparatively short time, the students will be of more help the more they learn about the work. Orientation classes are held to acquaint them with the different departments and with the purposes of the hospital.

With this addition to the nursing staff the number of employees is brought up almost to normal which should enable us to meet the high standards of nursing care that we have set for the N. S. H.

Seen here is the first issue of *The Stylus*, Norwich State Hospital's first newsletter, dated July 1941. *The Stylus* ran until November 1944. The newsletter was designed with a two-fold purpose. It kept the entire institution abreast of new changes and current happenings and also gave insight to members of the surrounding community of the hospital's work such as treatment programs and promoted events such as baseball games, field days, and holiday celebrations. The hospital's active community involvement during World War II was a frequently discussed topic. Patients had their own column, which they filled with poems and prose, along with ward club and party announcements. (Courtesy of Connecticut State Library.)

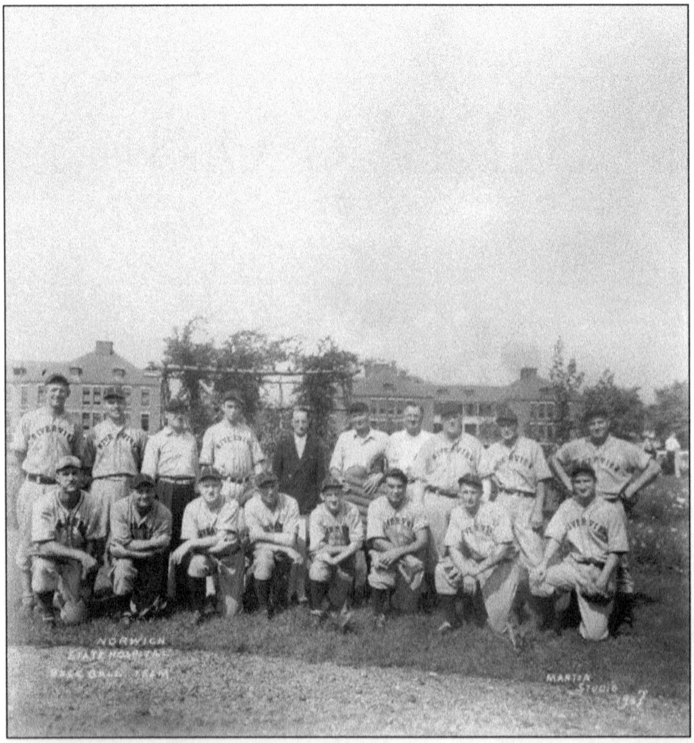

Baseball games had been a long running source of entertainment for both the staff and patients since the inception of Norwich State Hospital. Pictured here is the hospital's baseball team, the Riverview Team, on the hospital grounds in 1937. The Riverview Team played against other local teams, such as the widely known Electric Boat in Groton. Softball teams also existed among patients in different wards. The games were highly enjoyed by all, and game coverage was a running feature in *The Stylus*. (Author's collection.)

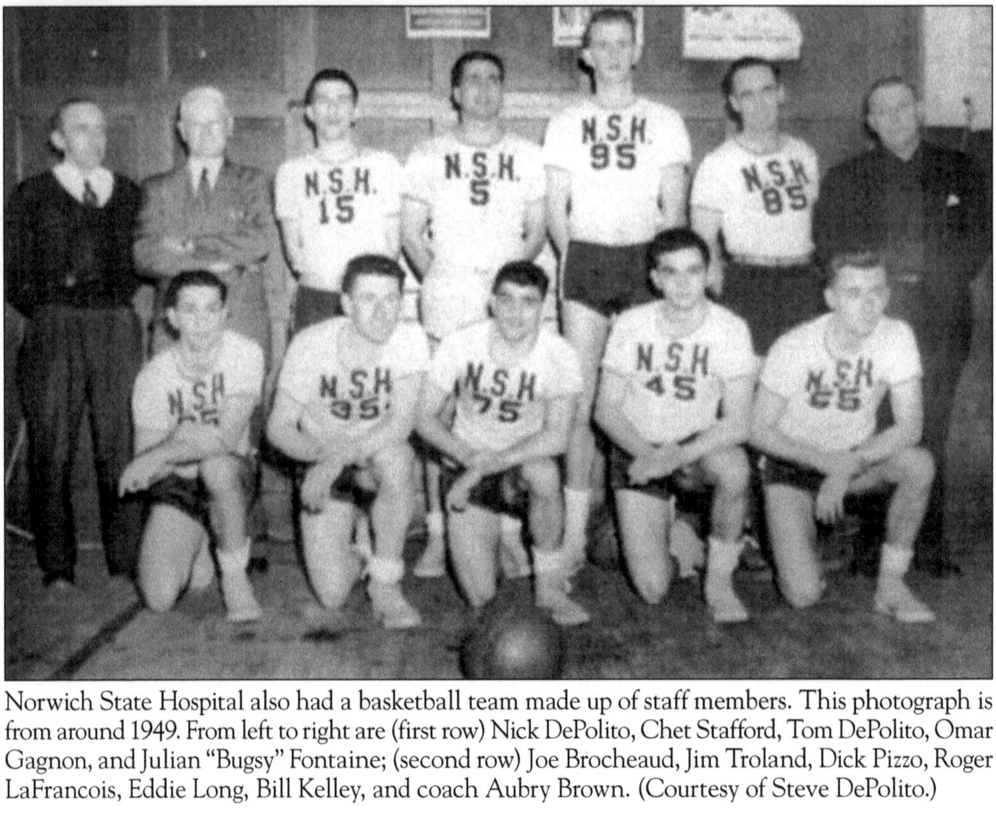

Norwich State Hospital also had a basketball team made up of staff members. This photograph is from around 1949. From left to right are (first row) Nick DePolito, Chet Stafford, Tom DePolito, Omar Gagnon, and Julian "Bugsy" Fontaine; (second row) Joe Brocheaud, Jim Troland, Dick Pizzo, Roger LaFrancois, Eddie Long, Bill Kelley, and coach Aubry Brown. (Courtesy of Steve DePolito.)

Pictured here are the cover (right) and two pages (below) of the Christmas program that was distributed throughout the hospital and community in 1940. Holidays were always celebrated at Norwich State Hospital. A plethora of activities for patients were scheduled each year, along with a grand Christmas dinner. Christmas carols were sung and holiday plays were held along with religious services in the grand auditorium. Memos were sent from the hospital to friends and relatives, encouraging them to send in gifts from home for their loved ones. Each year, Norwich State Hospital reached out to the community for gift donations for those patients who did not have family or loved ones at home. No patient was to be forgotten at Christmas. Staff frequently purchased and provided gifts for their patients themselves. (Both, author's collection.)

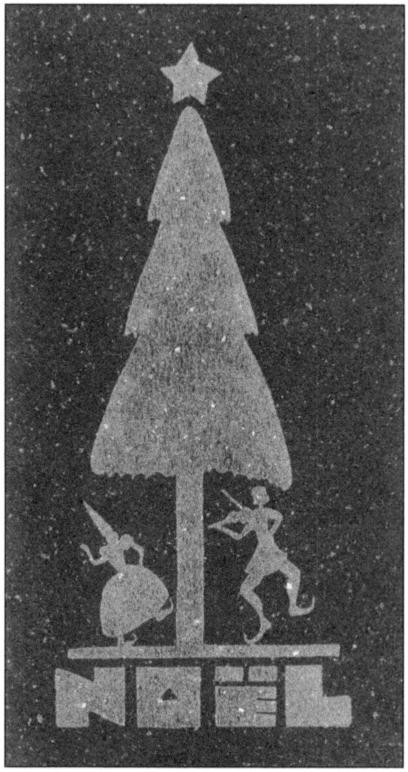

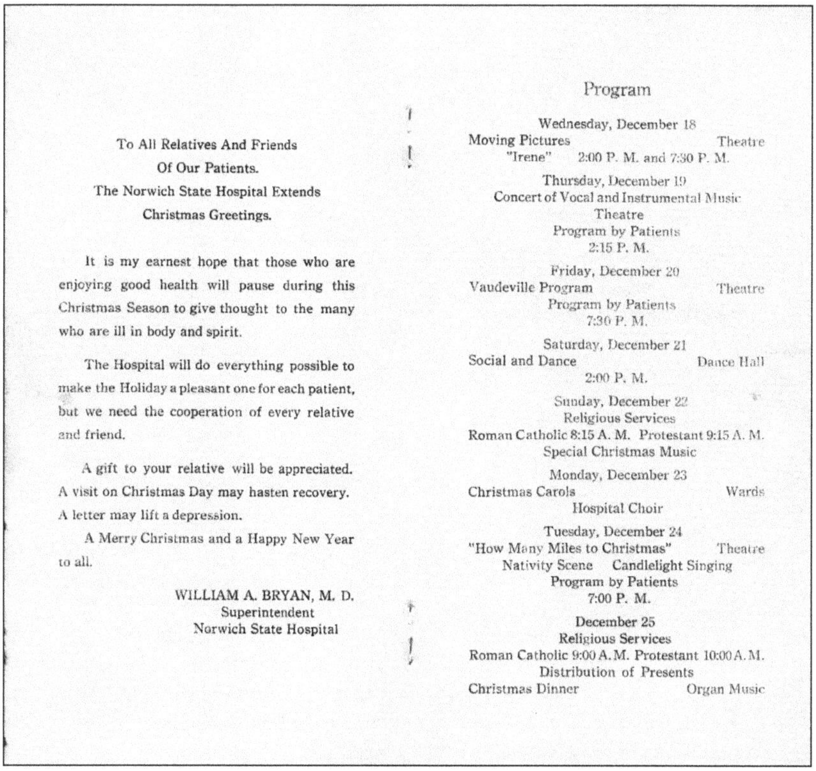

To All Relatives And Friends
Of Our Patients.
The Norwich State Hospital Extends
Christmas Greetings.

It is my earnest hope that those who are enjoying good health will pause during this Christmas Season to give thought to the many who are ill in body and spirit.

The Hospital will do everything possible to make the Holiday a pleasant one for each patient, but we need the cooperation of every relative and friend.

A gift to your relative will be appreciated.
A visit on Christmas Day may hasten recovery.
A letter may lift a depression.

A Merry Christmas and a Happy New Year to all.

WILLIAM A. BRYAN, M. D.
Superintendent
Norwich State Hospital

Program

Wednesday, December 18
Moving Pictures — Theatre
"Irene" 2:00 P. M. and 7:30 P. M.

Thursday, December 19
Concert of Vocal and Instrumental Music
Theatre
Program by Patients
2:15 P. M.

Friday, December 20
Vaudeville Program — Theatre
Program by Patients
7:30 P. M.

Saturday, December 21
Social and Dance — Dance Hall
2:00 P. M.

Sunday, December 22
Religious Services
Roman Catholic 8:15 A. M. Protestant 9:15 A. M.
Special Christmas Music

Monday, December 23
Christmas Carols — Wards
Hospital Choir

Tuesday, December 24
"How Many Miles to Christmas" — Theatre
Nativity Scene Candlelight Singing
Program by Patients
7:00 P. M.

December 25
Religious Services
Roman Catholic 9:00 A. M. Protestant 10:00 A. M.
Distribution of Presents
Christmas Dinner — Organ Music

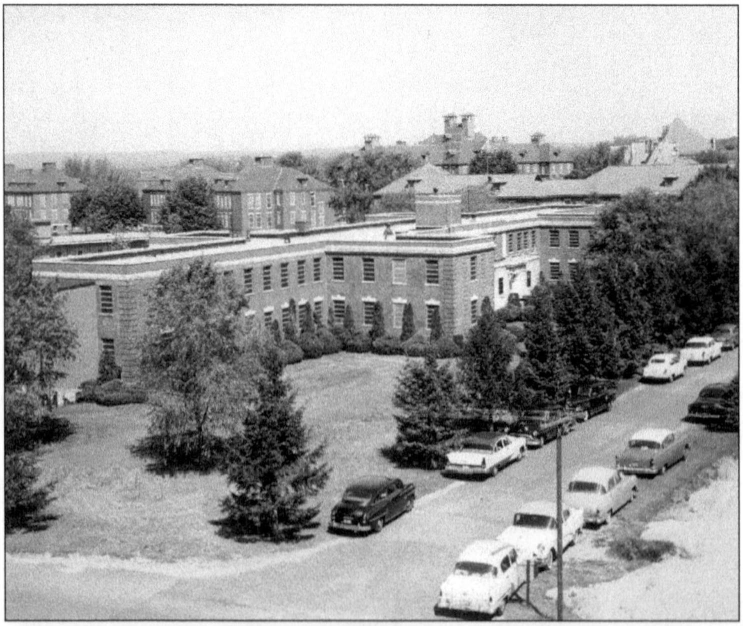

On the cusp of Dr. Bryan's new superintendence, 1939 also saw the addition of new buildings. Another new employees' home was erected and a new tuberculosis hospital, Seymour (pictured here around 1950), was constructed to replace the old dilapidated and unsafe Pines building. Seymour was named for Origen S. Seymour, a member of the hospital's board of trustees. (Courtesy of Brian Girasoli.)

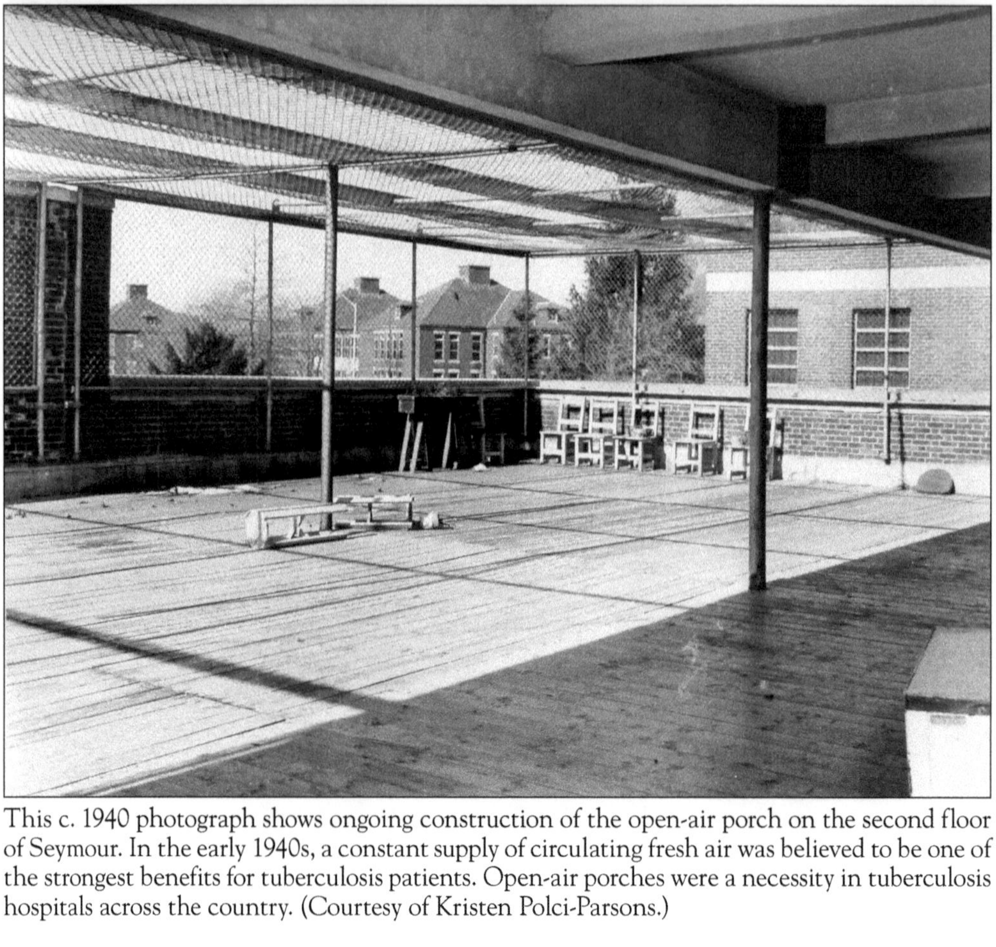

This c. 1940 photograph shows ongoing construction of the open-air porch on the second floor of Seymour. In the early 1940s, a constant supply of circulating fresh air was believed to be one of the strongest benefits for tuberculosis patients. Open-air porches were a necessity in tuberculosis hospitals across the country. (Courtesy of Kristen Polci-Parsons.)

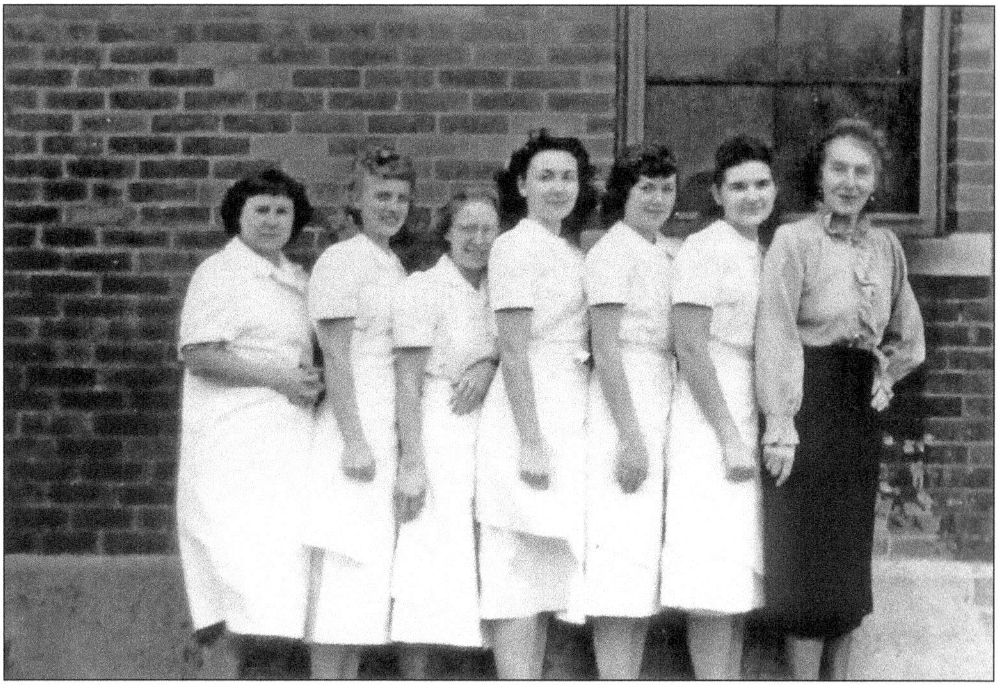

Laboratory services that had been previously neglected flourished under Dr. Bryan's new command. The photograph above from the mid-1940s shows Norwich State Hospital's laboratory staff posed outside the laboratory building. Lab techs from left to right are Medora Mitten, Ann MacDonald, Mary R. Risch, Nancy Bullard Kern, Mary Mellor Rathbone, Lillian Karkutt Schaeffer, and Dr. Hannah Pierson. MacDonald began her laboratory career in the mid-1940s at Norwich State Hospital and retired 40 years later. The laboratory building is pictured below in 1931. (Above, courtesy of Ann MacDonald; below, courtesy of Preston Historical Society.)

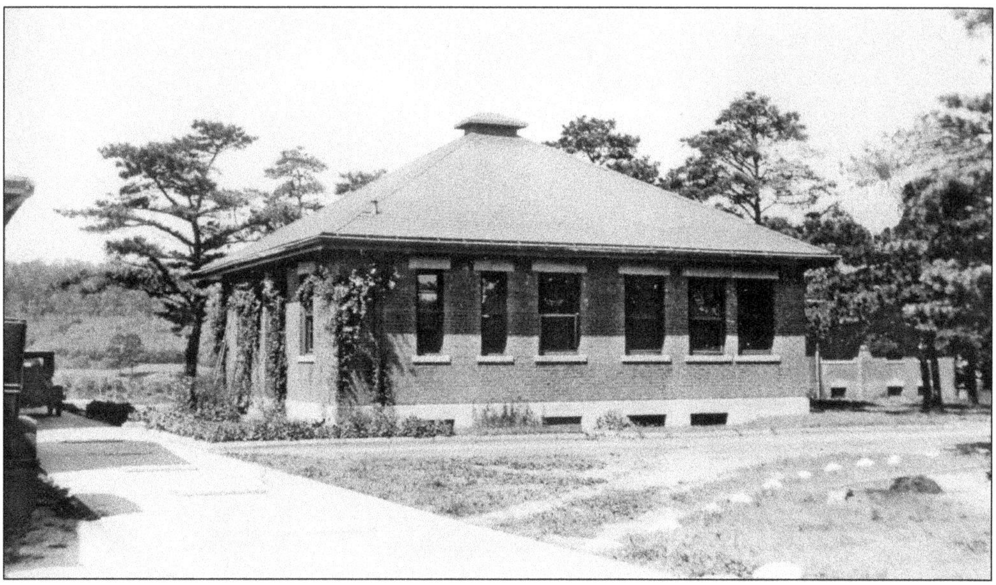

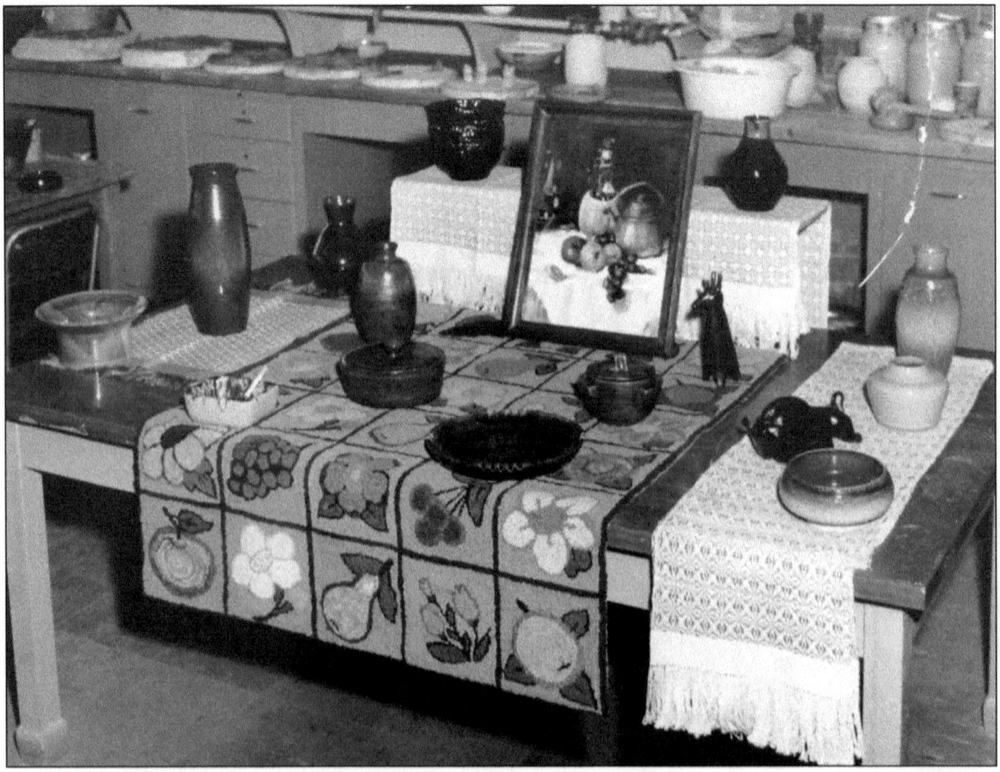

Dr. Bryan initiated cleanup campaigns on all the wards and insisted that articles made by the patients no longer be sold to the public, but used on the wards to make them more attractive, comfortable, and homelike. Dr. Bryan was considered revolutionary in his belief that homelike surroundings were conducive to the patients' comfort, happiness, and chance of recovery. Thirty years after Dr. Bryan's concept was implemented, the Joint Commission on Accreditation of Hospitals emphasized the importance of homelike surroundings in psychiatric hospital wards nationwide. The photographs on this page show many of the handmade items patients crafted at Norwich State Hospital. (Both, courtesy of Kristen Polci-Parsons.)

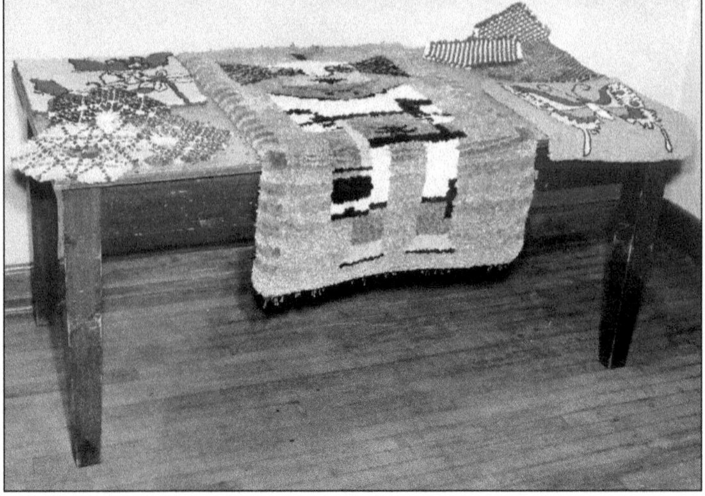

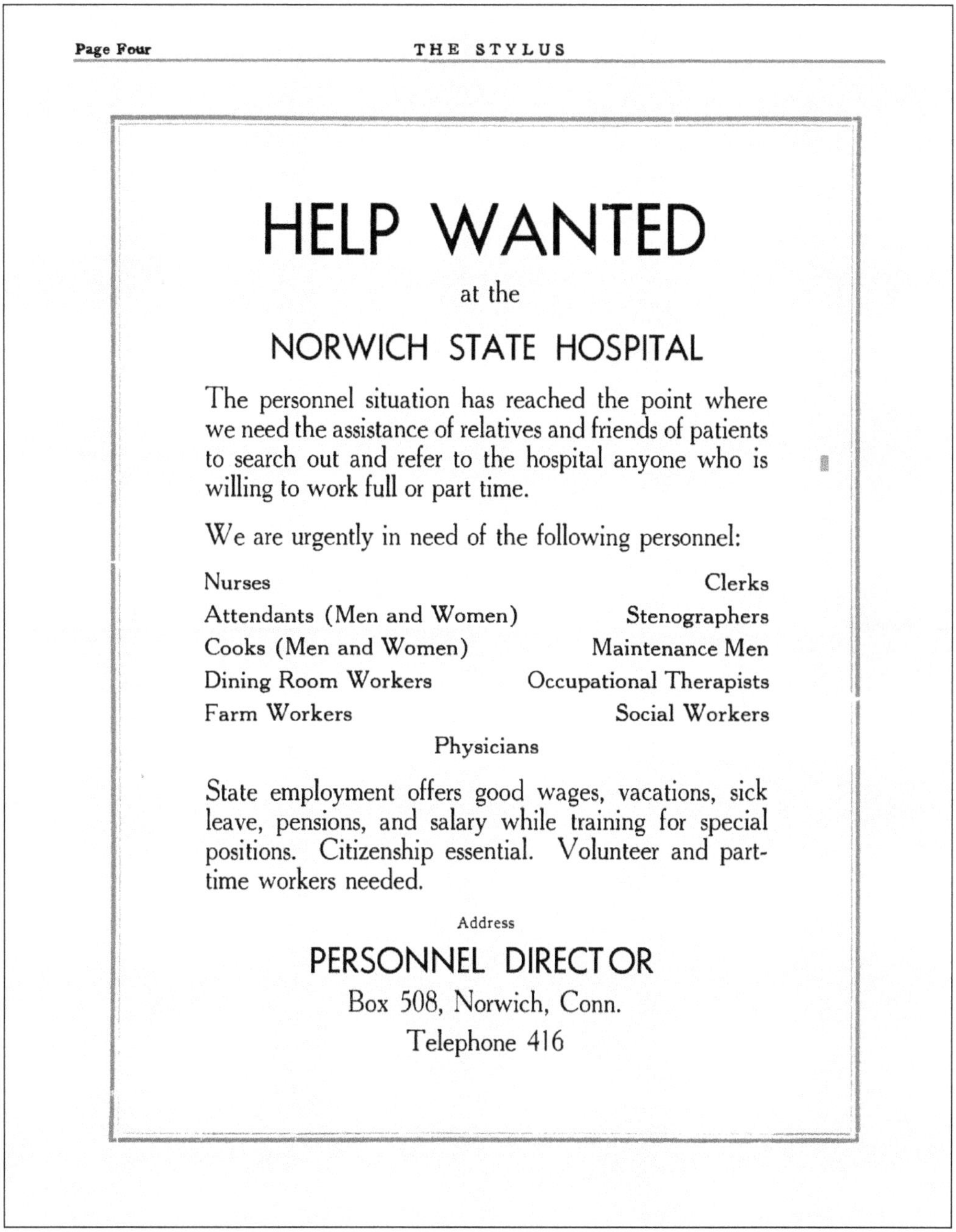

Page Four THE STYLUS

HELP WANTED

at the

NORWICH STATE HOSPITAL

The personnel situation has reached the point where we need the assistance of relatives and friends of patients to search out and refer to the hospital anyone who is willing to work full or part time.

We are urgently in need of the following personnel:

Nurses	Clerks
Attendants (Men and Women)	Stenographers
Cooks (Men and Women)	Maintenance Men
Dining Room Workers	Occupational Therapists
Farm Workers	Social Workers
Physicians	

State employment offers good wages, vacations, sick leave, pensions, and salary while training for special positions. Citizenship essential. Volunteer and part-time workers needed.

Address

PERSONNEL DIRECTOR

Box 508, Norwich, Conn.

Telephone 416

This help wanted ad from 1942 ran on the back page of *The Stylus* for nearly two years. Numerous physicians and staff left Norwich State Hospital to aid the wounded during World War II. The practice of employing college students as attendants and high school teachers who were interested in gaining experience working with the mentally ill was one solution Dr. Bryan found to the manpower problem. Wartime staffing shortages also took many competent patients from their wards and gave them positions as patient attendants. These methods of combatting the staffing shortage were considered unusual at the time but had a positive impact on the hospital. Many of the patient attendants did so well that they were later employed by the hospital. (Courtesy of Connecticut State Library.)

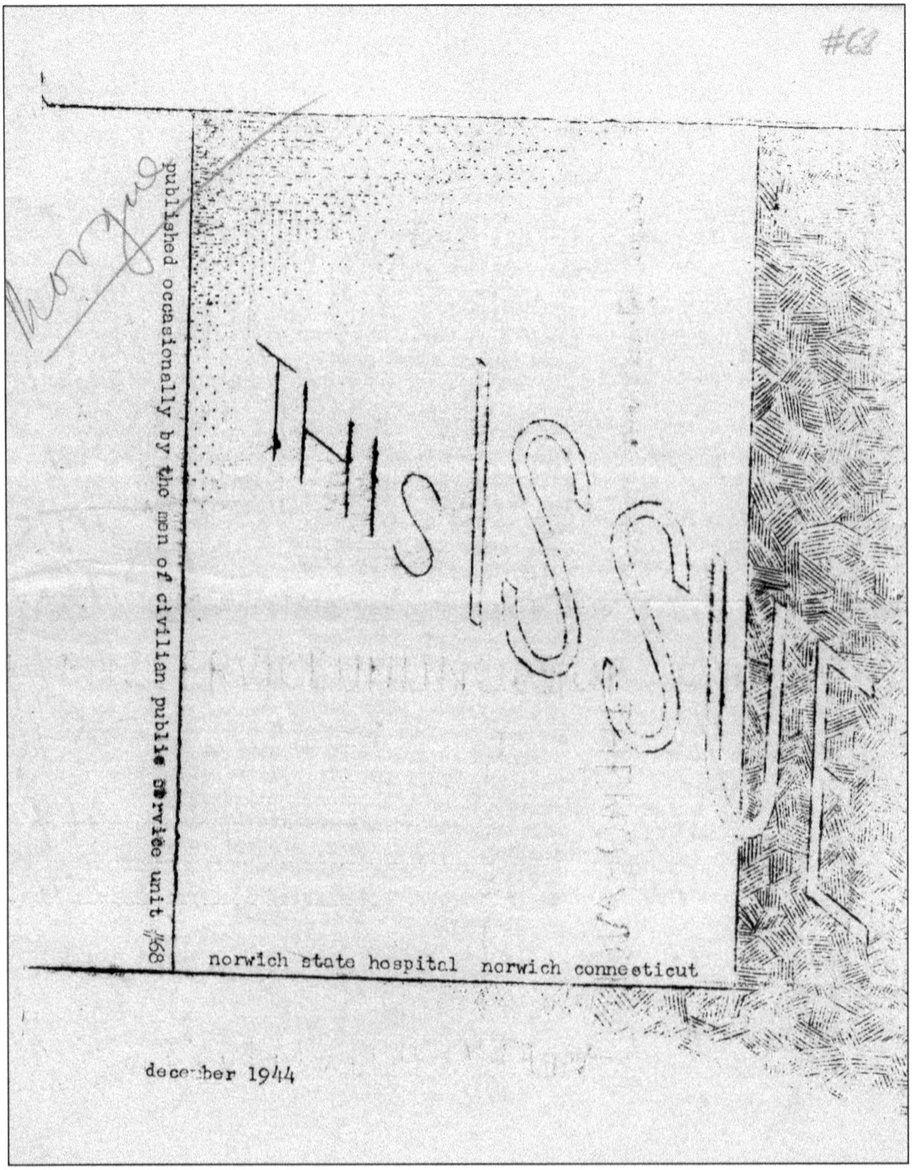

Dr. Bryan also recruited conscientious objectors to supplement staff during this critical time. This was a common practice by state hospitals throughout the country during World War II. Pictured is the cover of a newsletter from 1944 the conscientious objectors (COs) maintained throughout their service at Norwich State Hospital. COs expressed varied reasons for refusing to fight in the war. Many of them were members of pacifist church groups. The first group of COs arrived at Norwich in December 1942 and consisted of 27 men from Michigan. In 1943, a total of 47 COs were assigned to the hospital under the joint direction of Selective Service and the United Brethren Service Committee. Norwich State Hospital was designated as Civilian Public Service Unit No. 68. The COs primarily worked as attendants. The service of COs nationwide led to the founding of the National Mental Health Foundation, an organization established by young COs who succeeded in exposing the poor conditions and disgusting physical abuses they discovered in state hospitals throughout the country. (Courtesy of Civilian Public Service Camps Newsletters, Swarthmore College Peace Collection.)

Mothers of Soldiers

Mothers of men who have heard the call
You have given your sons, your very all
Each stalwart son in the thick of the fray
Is guarding our shores from the tyrant's sway.

Blue eyed Johnny seems only a boy,
We know that you cherish his very first toy
It seems only yesterday you heard his prayers,
And tucked him to bed safely upstairs.

Dear little mothers of sons in the fray
We know your fears from day to day
We know your heartache, we know your tears,
We know your inmost heartbreaking fears.
We know your valor, we know your worth.
Dearest of all little mothers on earth.

R. K. G., Woodward Building.

* * *

The fears patients exhibited during World War II seemed more about their loved ones than themselves, as seen in this poem from a 1943 issue of *The Stylus*. Dr. Bryan ensured that the hospital took every necessary precaution because of the hospital's proximity to the US Navy submarine base in Groton, just nine miles away. Blackout curtains were made by patients and air-raid drills were conducted regularly. The hospital only saw one real air-raid warning. (Courtesy of Connecticut State Library.)

Return Postage Guaranteed, Box 508, Norwich, Conn. Sec. 562, P. L. & R.

THE STYLUS

OF

THE NORWICH STATE HOSPITAL, NORWICH, CONN.

Vol. 4 NOVEMBER, 1944 No. 11

IN MEMORIAM: WILLIAM A. BRYAN, M. D.

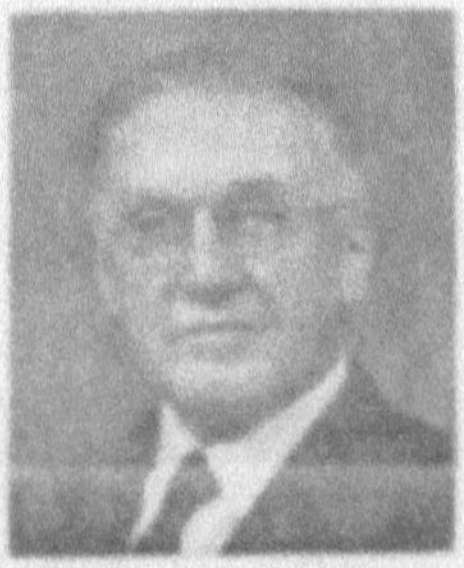

With the death of Dr. William Alvin Bryan on November 7, 1944, the field of Psychiatry was deprived of one of its outstanding pioneers in mental hospital administration.

Dr. Bryan was born in Creston, Iowa, on November 21, 1883. He received his M. D. degree at George Washington University in 1908, served as interne in the United States Public Health Service in Chelsea, Massachusetts from 1909 to 1910, and then became Assistant Physician at the Clarinda (Iowa) State Hospital from 1910 to 1912, the Cherokee (Iowa) State Hospital from 1912 to 1916, and the Boston Psychopathic Hospital from 1916 to 1917. From 1917 to 1920 he was Assistant Superintendent of the Danvers Hospital and from 1920 to 1921 assistant to the Commissioner of the Department of Mental Diseases in Massachusetts. Most of his professional life (1921 to 1940) was spent as Superintendent of the Worcester State Hospital. In May, 1940, he became Superintendent of the Norwich State Hospital.

From 1933 to 1937 he was Lecturer in Social Administration at Boston University, and in 1942 he was appointed Lecturer in Psychiatry and Mental Hygiene with the rank of Clinical Professor at the Yale University School of Medicine.

The psychiatric point-of-view which Dr. Bryan advanced throughout all his years as an administrator is summarized in this statement from his book, "Administrative Psychiatry," published in 1936: "It becomes increasingly evident that the future of psychiatry and its influence on public health will be built around the hospital." This philosophy gave substance to the many plans with which he was always engaged. He always had his eyes on the future and was frequently criticized for being visionary. These criticisms usually melted away with the realization of projects previously considered impossible. He was a man of fire. His persistence in fighting for his ideas found concrete expression in the establishment of the Schizophrenia Research Unit at the Worcester State Hospital and in the establishment of an extensive teaching program at both Worcester and Norwich.

Once convinced of the worth of his ideas, he did not fail to recognize the need of assistance for which he asked without embarrassment. Having picked the men and women to assist in his programs, he defended them loyally and asked only that they do the work of which he knew them to be capable. He was always open to new ideas.

He was a curious mixture of patience in working toward a far-distant goal and impatience in carrying out an idea which he felt was good. Remonstrances that conditions were not yet ripe for a particular program were almost invariably met with the retort, "The idea should be put into effect and the conditions will ripen of themselves."

He was not without insight into his own personality and often referred to what he called his "impulsiveness," which his associates recognized as intolerance of the lazy, the unimaginative and the incompetent. His high distinction as an administrator was in part due to the fact that he demanded the best efforts of everyone who worked for him.

His personal courage, especially in the last year of his life—when lesser men would have succumbed to the harassing exigencies of war-time conditions and failing health—is an inspiration to those of us who knew him.

Most of all he was concerned with the future of psychiatry in terms of the community's attitude toward mental hospitals. He wrote: "When people understand that their relatives and friends must be cared for by experienced and well-trained individuals and that the encroachment of partisan politics into hospital administration takes its toll in a lessened chance for recovery of the patient, this practice will cease. But the responsibility of educating the community belongs to the administrator."

Dr. Bryan died believing in the

(Continued on Page 4, Column 3)

Due to the wartime paper shortage, *The Stylus* was discontinued in November 1944 after this final issue honored Dr. Bryan. Dr. Bryan lost his battle with ill health and died at his home on the Norwich State Hospital grounds on November 7, 1944. He was hailed as a pioneer in administrative psychiatry. He had many advanced ideas to improve psychiatry and the state hospital and never hesitated to implement them. His dedication to his work and his hospital was untiring. The high standards he held Norwich State Hospital to led to accreditation by the American Medical Association and the American Psychiatric Association. Despite his declining health in the last year of his life, he courageously led Norwich State Hospital through the difficulties of World War II. His legacy was memorialized in this last issue of *The Stylus* and his death was perceived as a tremendous loss not only to Norwich State Hospital, but to the field of psychiatry as a whole. (Courtesy of Connecticut State Library.)

Four

Norwich State Hospital on the International Map

Norwich State Hospital carried on Dr. Bryan's legacy as Dr. Riley H. Guthrie came from St. Elizabeth's Hospital in Washington, DC, and assumed superintendent duties on January 1, 1945. Dr. Guthrie was immediately faced with the continuing challenges of staff shortages, the ongoing increase in patient population, and inadequate security at the hospital's criminally insane building. In the wake of these challenges, Dr. Guthrie and Norwich State Hospital faced an unforeseen and catastrophic tragedy: the loss of Dr. Guthrie's wife, Anne Hoge Guthrie.

At 2:30 a.m. on Friday, April 30, 1948, Anne awoke to smoke and alerted her husband to a fire in their home on Norwich State Hospital grounds. Dr. Guthrie hurried downstairs to telephone the fire department, believing his wife was following close behind. Dr. Guthrie evacuated the home, thinking his wife was already safely outside. He searched for Anne but she was nowhere to be found. He returned to try to find her, but was overcome by dense smoke and forced to retreat back outside. Former Norwich firefighter Edward Angel, chief plant and maintenance engineer at NSH, heard the fire alarm from his home near the hospital. He responded to the fire and attempted to rescue Anne. Angel also could not brave the thick smoke and emerged from the home without her. He collapsed on the ground, repeating softly, "I can't find her." Mr. and Mrs. Horace Clay, also NSH employees, helped to carry Angel to the Lippitt Building, where he was pronounced dead due to smoke inhalation and cardiac arrest. The responding firefighters were also unable to rescue Anne. She was later found on the floor partially covered by an overturned table in a small dressing room off the bedroom she shared with her husband.

Dr. Guthrie resigned three months later due to ill health. Dr. Ronald H. Kettle, then assistant superintendent, took the lead as superintendent and transformed Norwich State Hospital into a polished, modern, and highly regarded psychiatric hospital during his administration. His superintendence brought many exciting new changes, including the hospital's third and final name change and the establishment of a new state-of-the-art therapeutic building that sparked international interest.

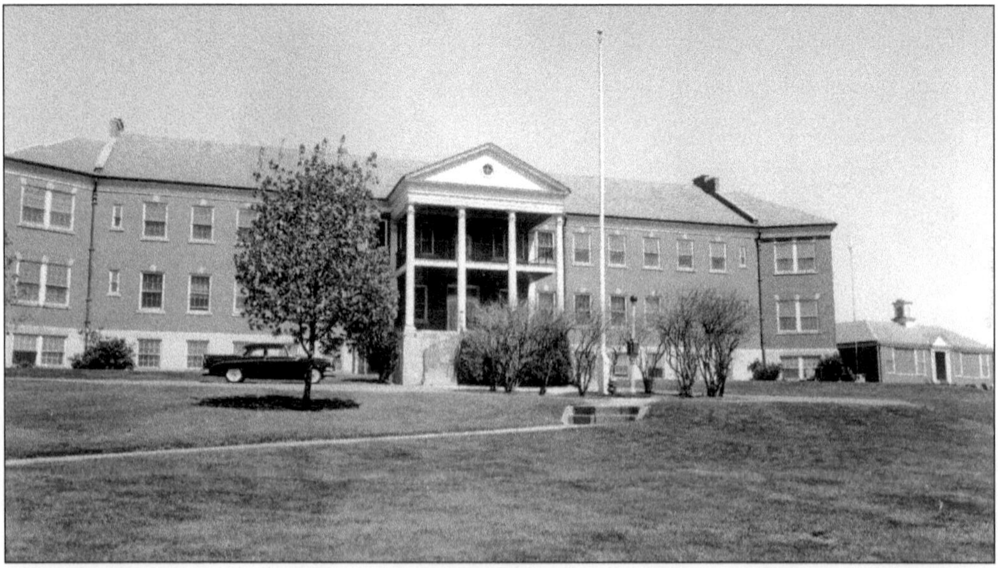

During World War II, Dr. Bryan had purchased the former New London County Home for tuberculosis patients with the expectation of repurposing it as a children's unit. Wartime shortages in building materials and personnel delayed the building's renovation. Under Dr. Guthrie's administration, the work was completed and the building was readied instead for 130 geriatric patients. The building was named in memory of Dr. William Bryan and opened with official dedication ceremonies on Friday, May 20, 1949. Shown here around 1950, the William A. Bryan Building was the first of more new buildings to join the Norwich State Hospital campus. (Courtesy of Brian Girasoli.)

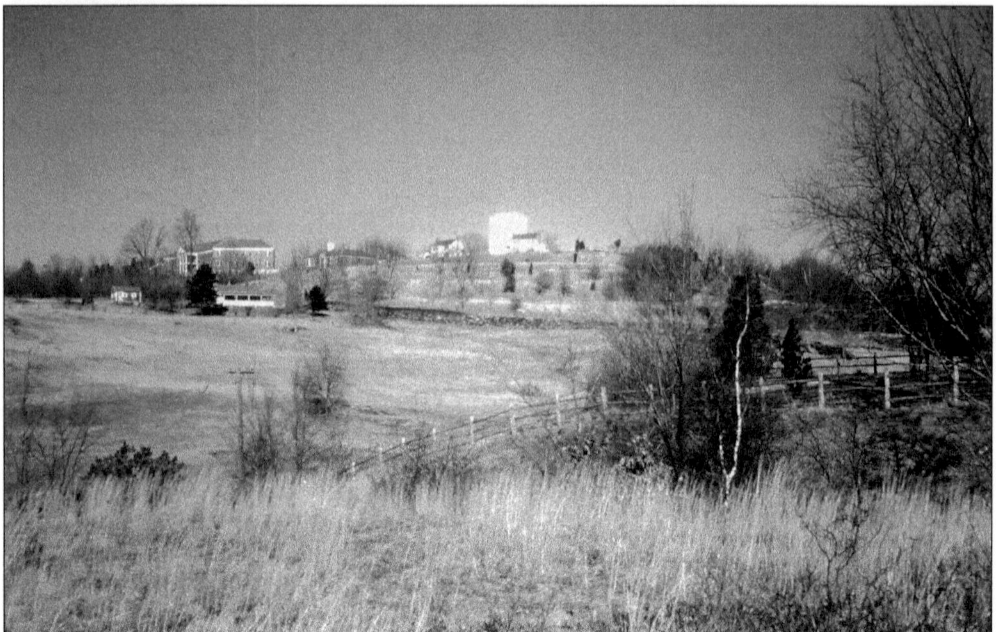

The Bryan Building, seen here around 1961, sat above Route 12 at the northern end of the hospital grounds. Behind the building stood what became known as Hospital Hill, an area of 14 cottages for physicians and their families who lived on NSH grounds. (Courtesy of Allan Burns.)

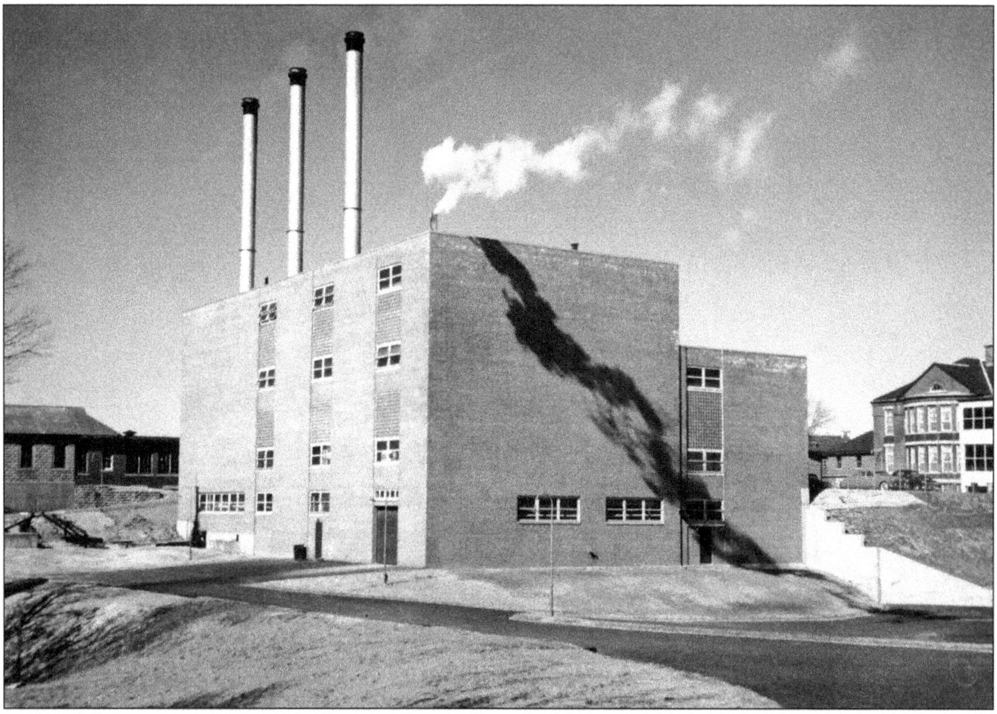

Under Dr. Kettle's administration, the 1950s were marked by a boom in building expansion at Norwich State Hospital. Eight different state-of-the-art buildings were erected over a period of 10 years. Among these were a new powerhouse (above) and laundry building (below), which were completed and serving the hospital well by 1952. The 1950s also saw the closure of older dilapidated buildings as the new structures went up. (Both, courtesy of Preston Historical Society.)

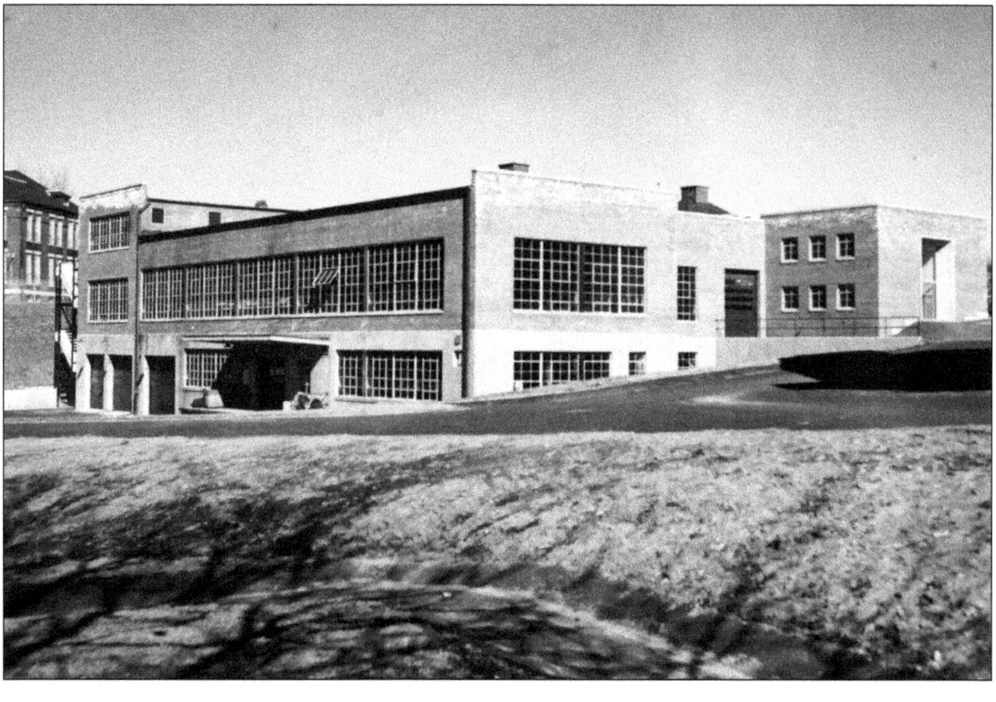

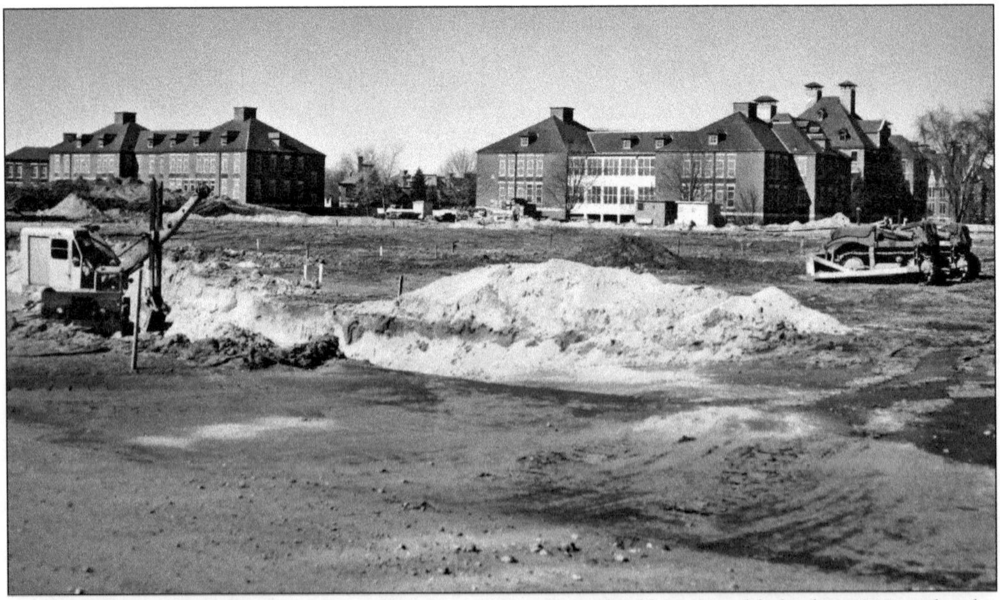

Norwich State Hospital's occupational therapy department had been established in 1921 under the direction of Harry Kromer. From that time, occupational therapy (OT) activities such as sewing, woodworking, and shoe repair were done in crude workshops scattered about the campus on the wards and in makeshift rooms in the basements of the ward buildings. During his superintendence, Dr. Guthrie wanted to centralize all OT programs in one building to boost their therapeutic progress and make organization significantly less difficult. This did not occur until nearly 10 years later under Dr. Kettle's administration. Grading for the new occupational therapy building began in 1953, pictured here. (Courtesy of Preston Historical Society.)

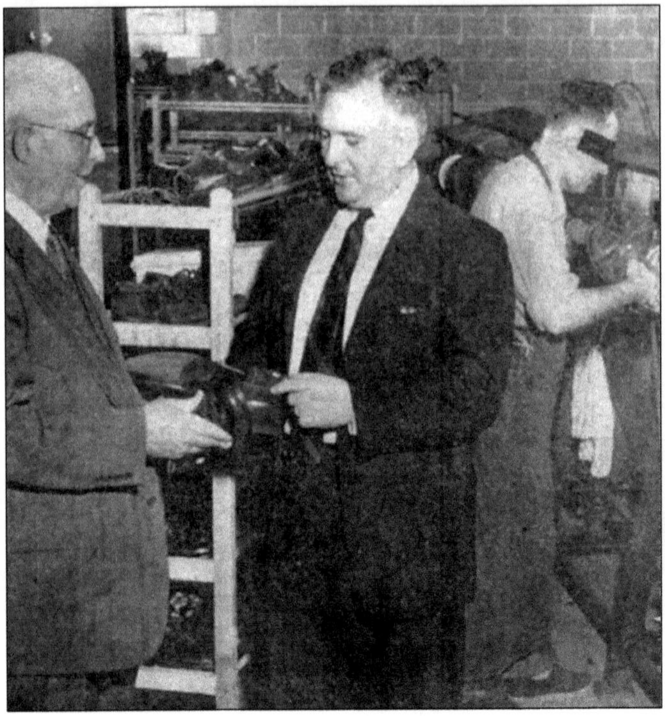

Harry Kromer (left) was regarded as one of the country's most outstanding specialists in occupational therapy. He ran Norwich State Hospital's OT department for over 40 years until his retirement. Many OT students from around the country traveled to Norwich State Hospital to study and learn from his methods. He is pictured here in 1956 showing high-quality shoe work done by the patients in the new OT building to David K. Boynick, Department of Mental Health staff. (Author's collection.)

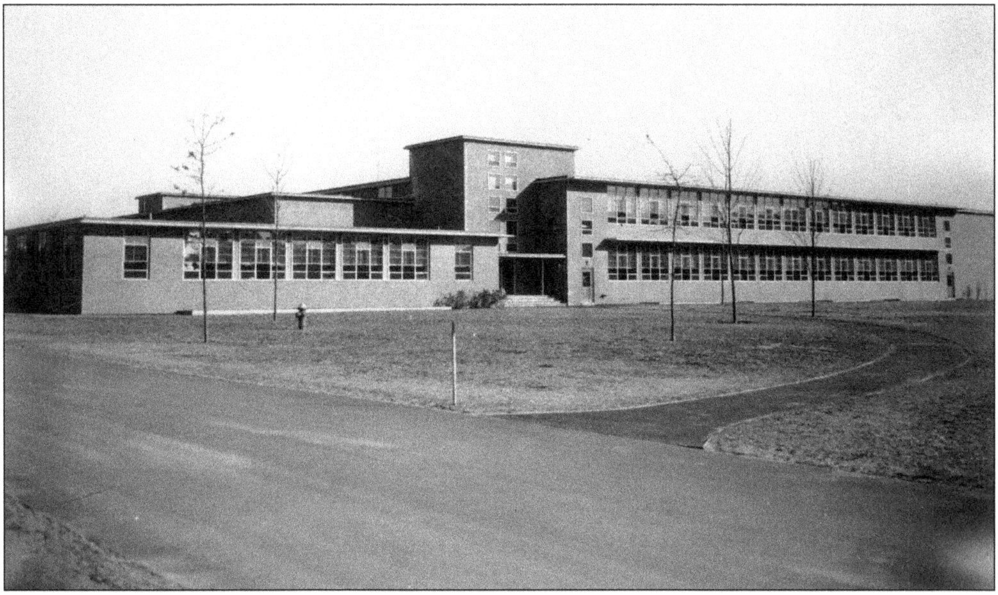

Dr. Kettle and his administration toured other mental hospitals in the country to gather ideas for Norwich State Hospital's new occupational therapy center. The hospitals they toured did not offer models that matched what they had in mind for NSH. Hartford architectural firm Ebbett, Frid and Prentice was hired to create the building they imagined. The building was completed and opened in 1956. The two-story Russell Occupational Therapy building placed NSH on the international map with its handsome new modern construction and large assortment of occupational therapies, all under one roof. Named for former hospital trustee chair Ruth Gardner Russell, the building was dedicated and formally opened with official ceremonies on March 10, 1956. Former Connecticut governor Abraham A. Ribicoff was ranking dignitary at the opening ceremonies. The unique unit attracted a great deal of attention and was frequently visited by psychiatrists from around the country and abroad. Two angles of the Russell Building's main entrance are seen here around 1956. (Both, courtesy of Brian Girasoli.)

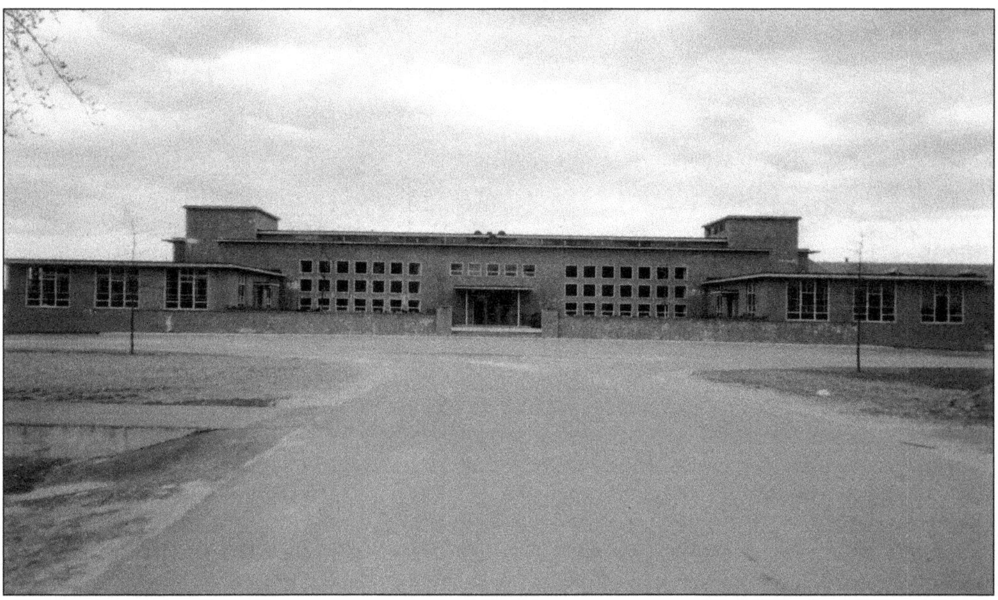

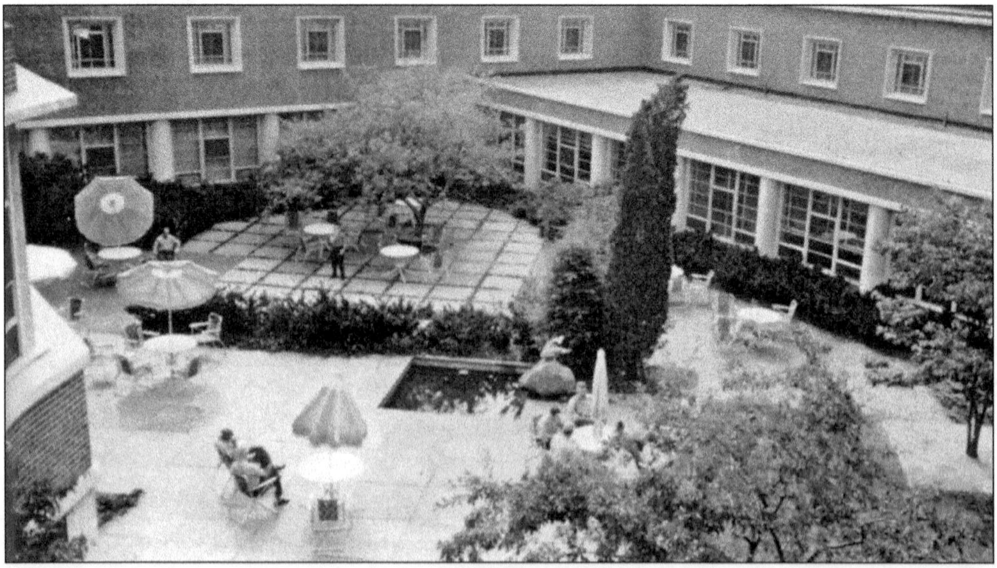

The hospital administration wanted the building to be designed more as a relaxing workshop and social center as opposed to an architectural monument. The focal point of the new center was its canteen, which opened into a large enclosed outdoor patio, pictured above in 1956. The patio was dotted with cheerfully colored umbrellas grouped around a small, shallow pool stocked with goldfish. The canteen and adjoining patio resembled a country club more than a psychiatric hospital. The Russell Building was purposely designed to provide an attractive, friendly atmosphere conducive to socialization. (Author's collection.)

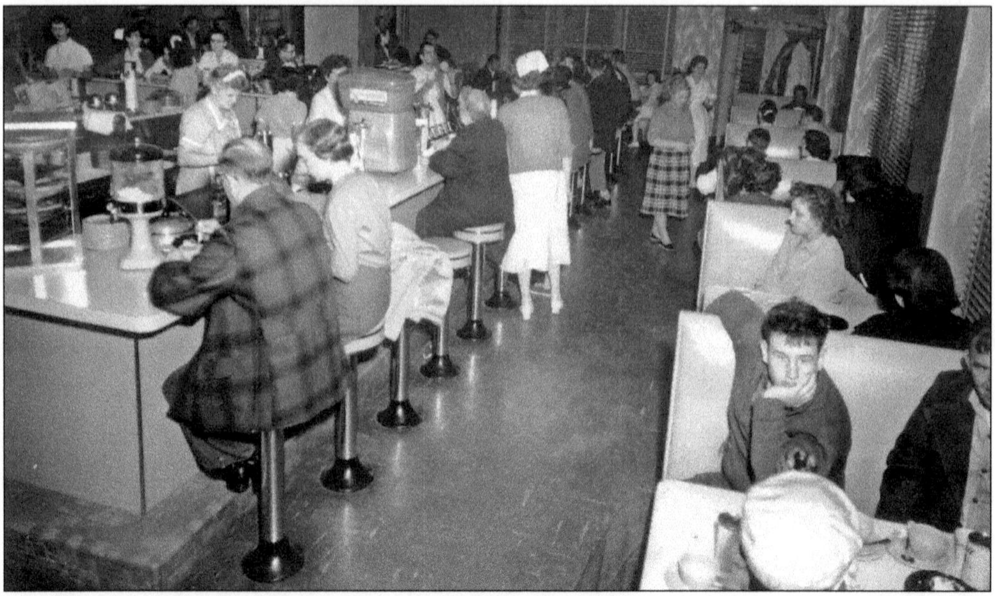

The canteen resembled a diner more than anything typically found in a mental hospital. It featured a snack bar and tables and booths. Light meals, coffee, and soda were served to patients, guests, and employees. Patients used the canteen almost as they would a regular restaurant. Hospital volunteers were often under the impression that the patients were completely unattended in the airy, free environment, but they were not. Attendants were always in the room but purposely made themselves as inconspicuous as possible. (Courtesy of Brian Girasoli.)

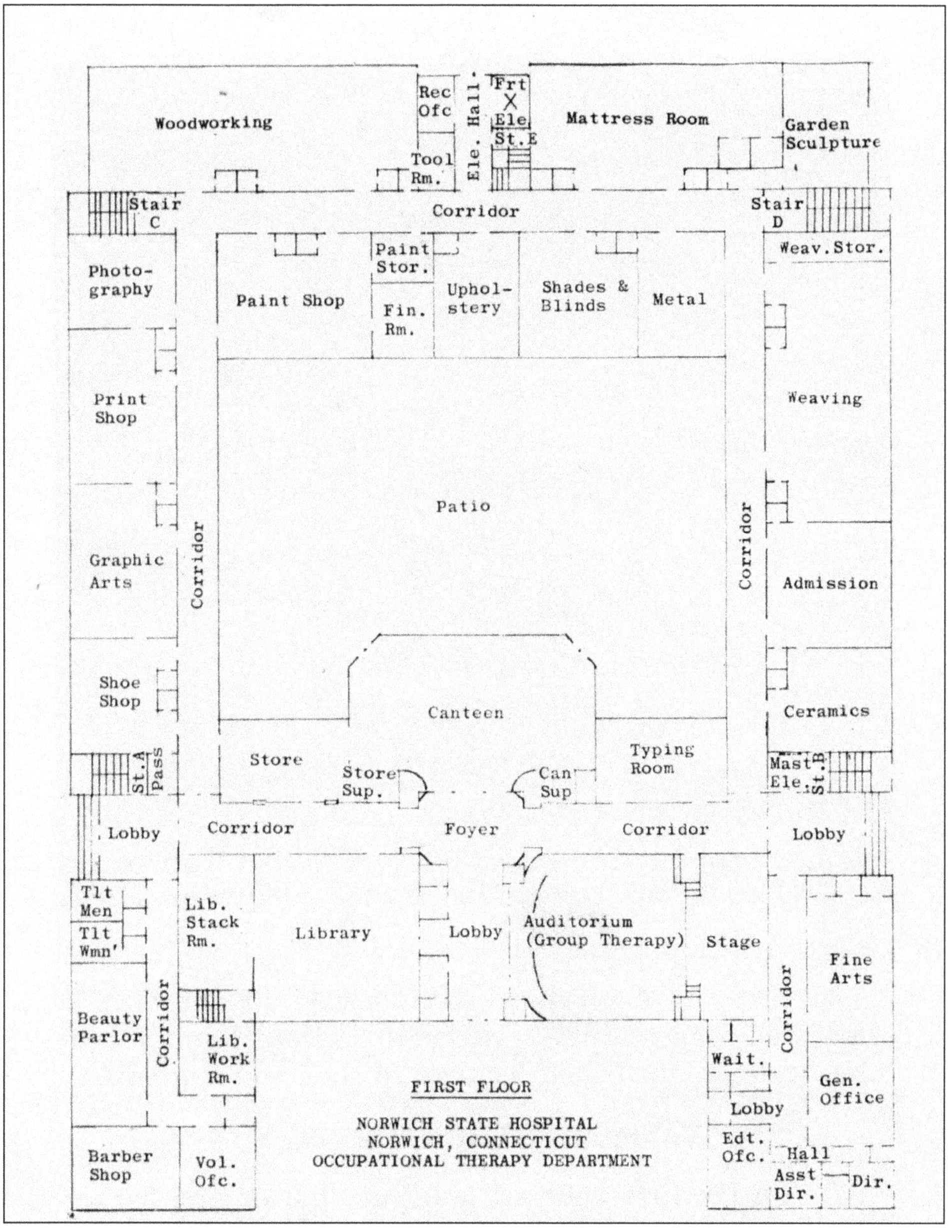

This layout of the Russell Building's ground floor shows a large portion of the variety of shops offered for therapeutic benefit. The ground floor contained large, well-lighted shops for woodworking, graphic arts, weaving, shoe repair, ceramics, painting, upholstery, and metalworking. The basement had large rooms for billiards, ping pong, shuffleboard, and a bowling alley. The canteen can be seen at the southern end of the open-air patio. Occupational therapy was an important department in state hospitals nationwide. OT programs took otherwise sedentary patients and gave them activities to focus on while building self-esteem in a social setting. Like other hospitals throughout the country, Norwich State Hospital's administration insisted that idle minds would not be apt to recover. In later years, occupational therapy was discontinued nationwide as a result of protests that patients' skills and labor were being taken advantage of by the state hospitals. (Author's collection.)

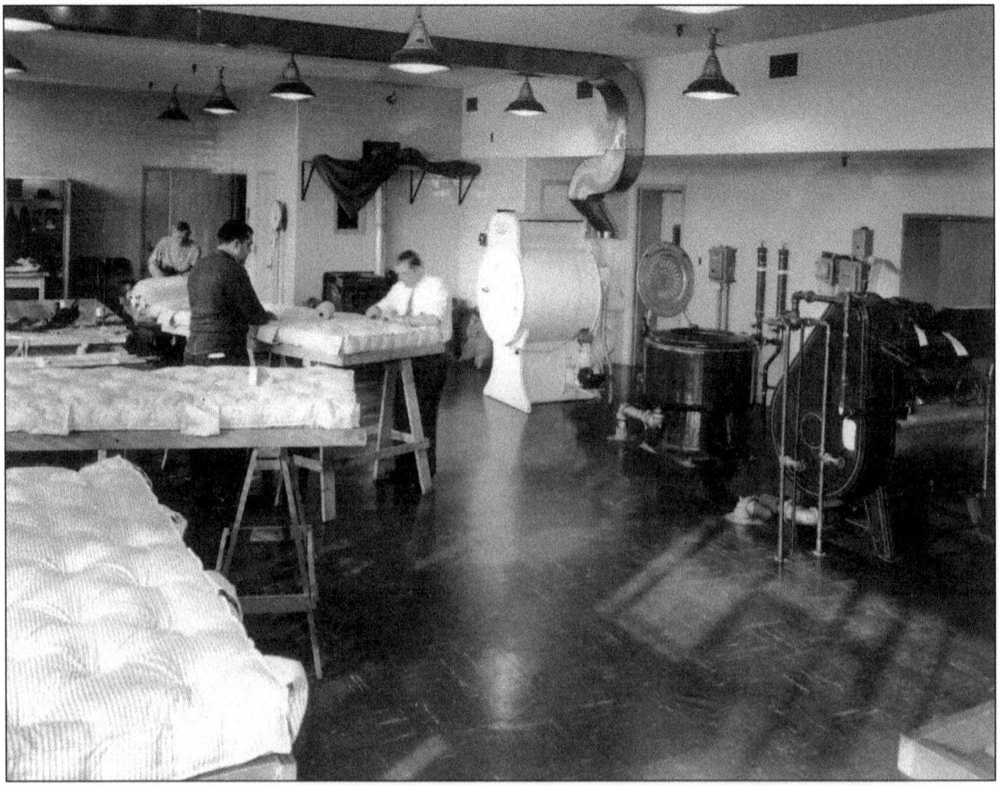

Shown here around 1956 is the mattress shop, where patients learned how to make and mend mattresses that were used on every ward of the hospital. The work patients did in shops like this would be misconstrued in later years as "free labor" at the advantage of the state hospital. This caused many occupational therapy shops to be discontinued. (Courtesy of Brian Girasoli.)

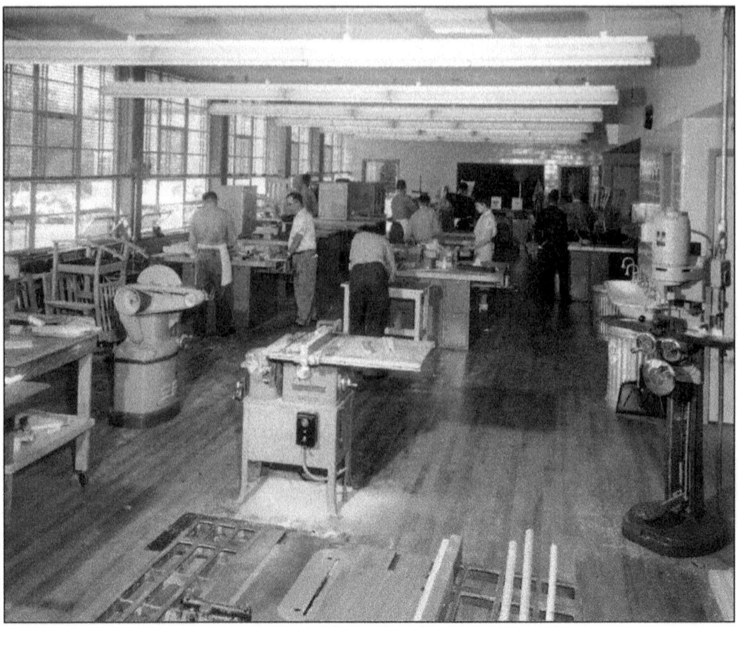

Male patients are seen here in the woodworking shop constructing furnishings such as small tables and chairs. Like many of the other shops in the occupational therapy building, the items made here were used among the wards. Patients enjoyed these workshops, as many of them were formerly employed in carpentry and woodworking careers before coming to the state hospital. (Courtesy of Brian Girasoli.)

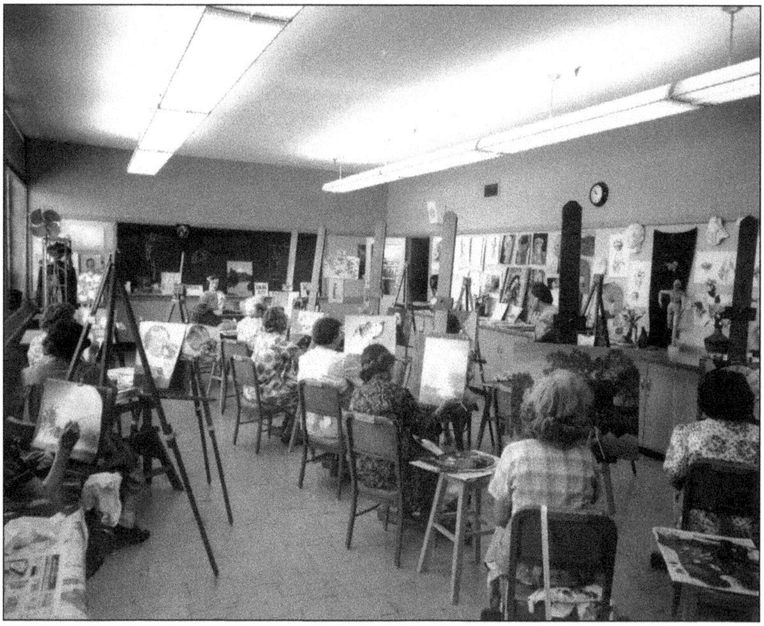

The painting and fine arts room on the first floor of the Russell Building is seen here appearing more like a college art classroom, with its blackboard and neatly arranged work areas, than what laymen would expect to see in a mental hospital. The patients create portraits and still life paintings in this c. 1956 photograph. (Courtesy of Brian Girasoli.)

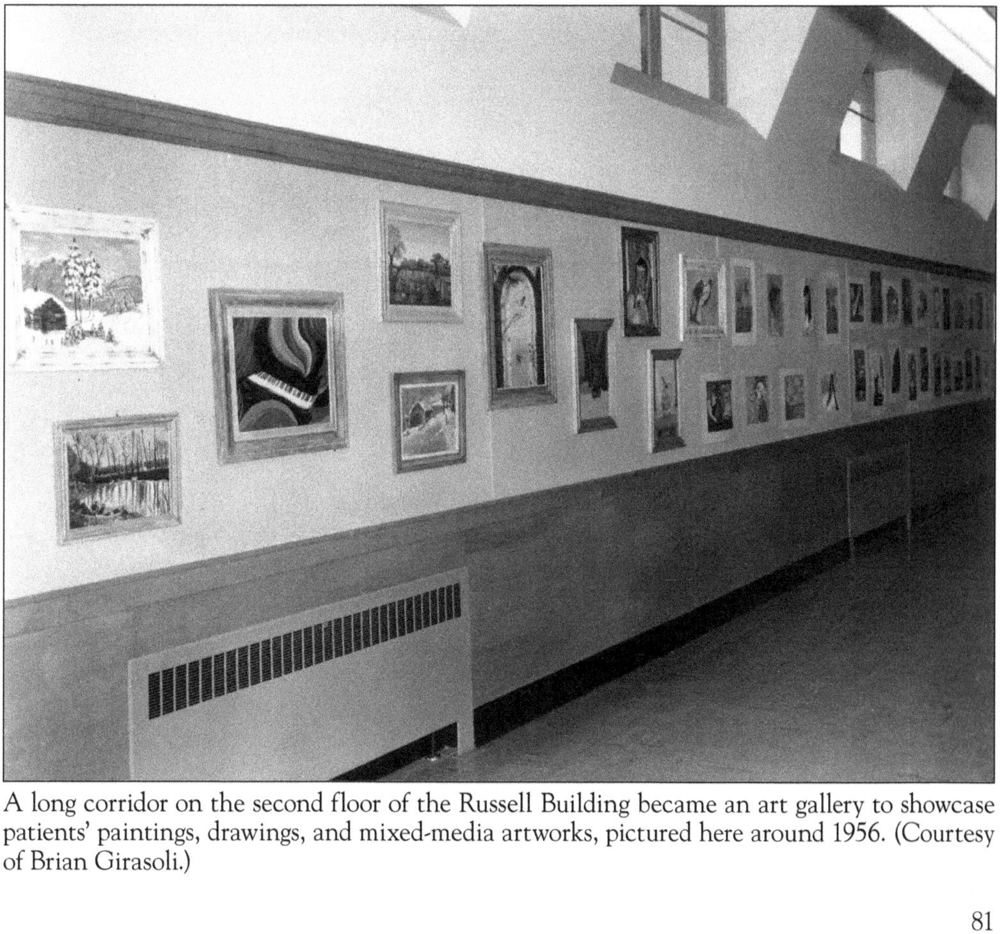

A long corridor on the second floor of the Russell Building became an art gallery to showcase patients' paintings, drawings, and mixed-media artworks, pictured here around 1956. (Courtesy of Brian Girasoli.)

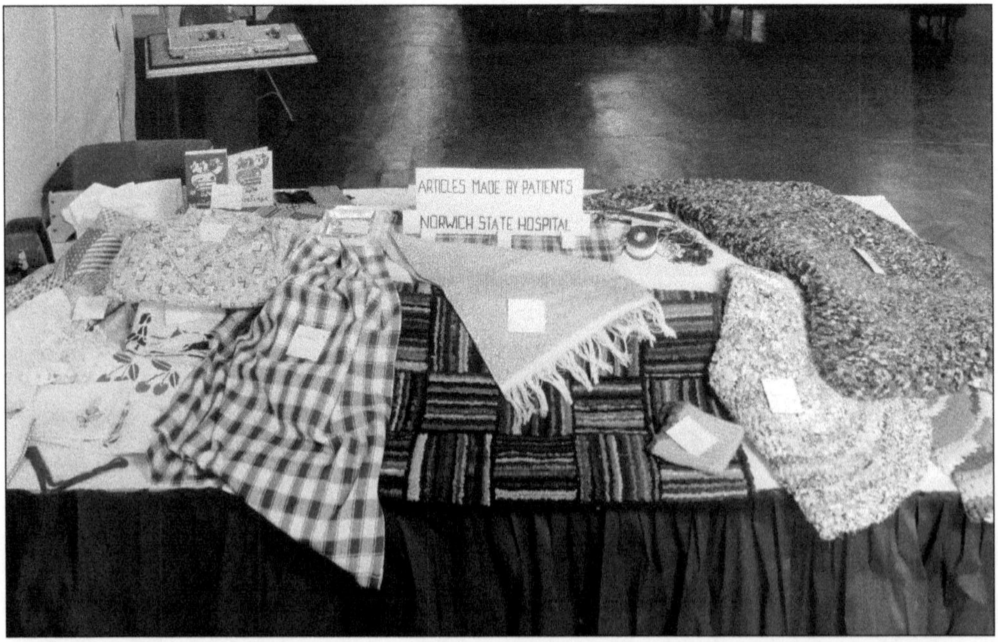

This photograph from 1957 shows many of the handmade articles patients created in the occupational therapy workshops. Various articles such as the garments and greeting cards pictured were displayed and sold at arts and crafts shows at the hospital and throughout the community. Note the small model of the Russell Building in the background. (Courtesy of Kristen Polci-Parsons.)

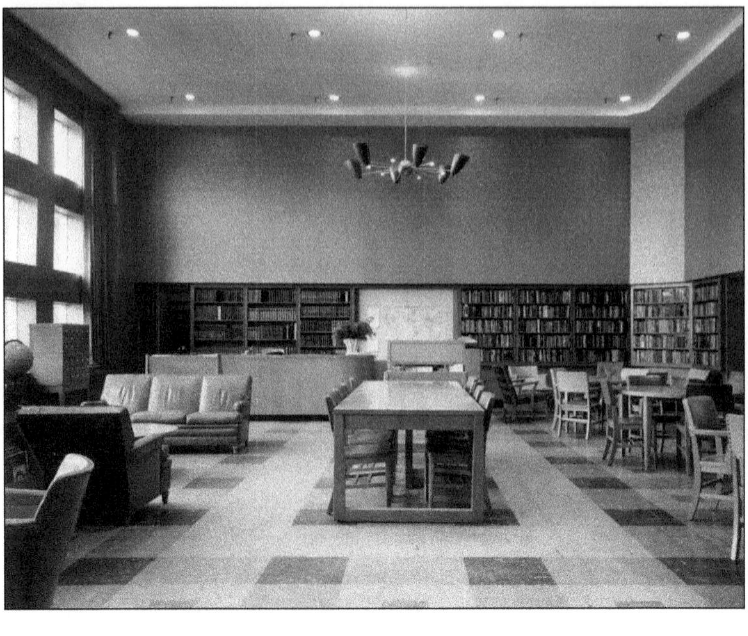

The Russell Building had a spacious and handsome library for patient use. The library had an excellent selection of books and magazines. Patients came every afternoon to relax in comfortable chairs and peruse as many books as they pleased. An average of 4,000 books were borrowed by patients each month. (Courtesy of Brian Girasoli.)

A large auditorium sat across the hall from the patients' library on the first floor. Dramatics, meetings, and lectures were held here. A group singing session conducted by volunteers is taking place in this c. 1956 photograph. (Courtesy of Brian Girasoli.)

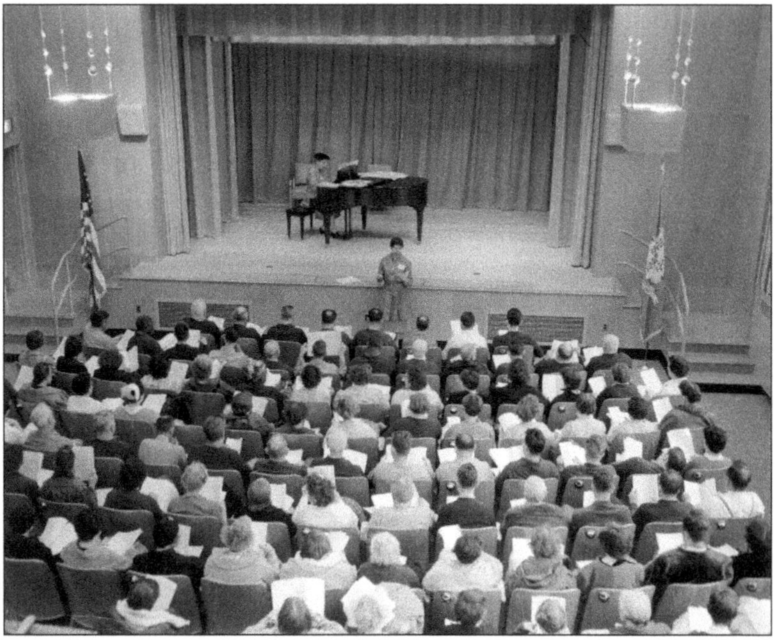

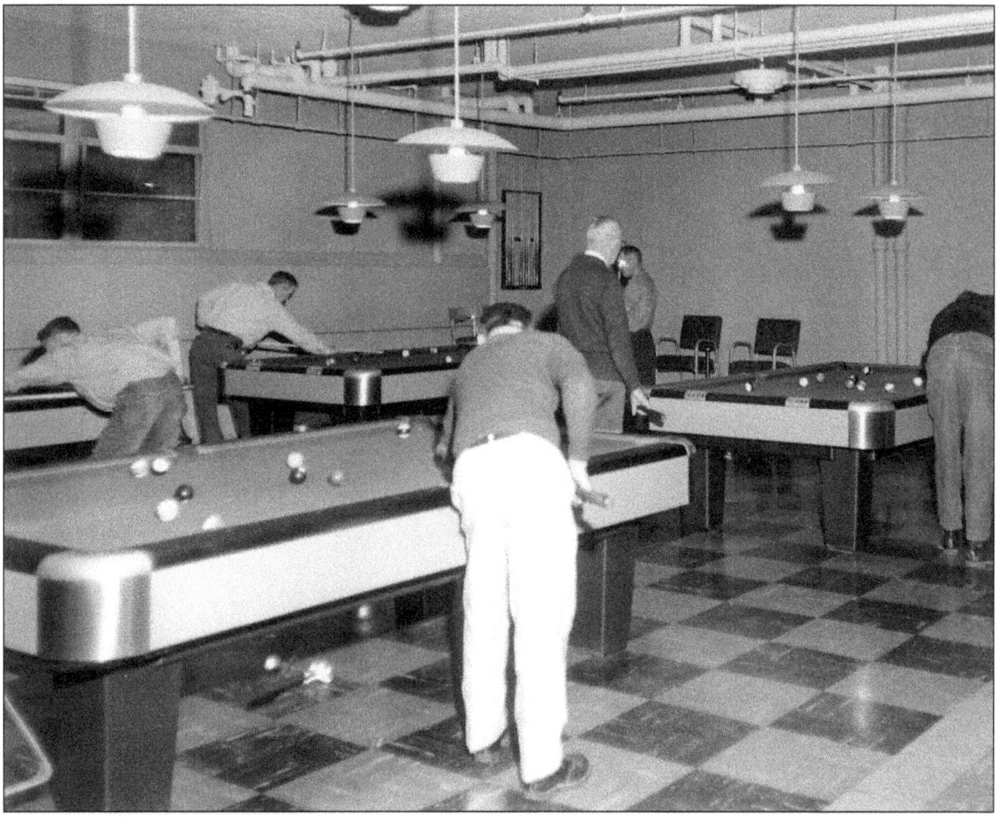

A large room for billiards sat near the bowling alley in the basement of the Russell Building. Games of billiards were greatly enjoyed by the patients. (Courtesy of Brian Girasoli.)

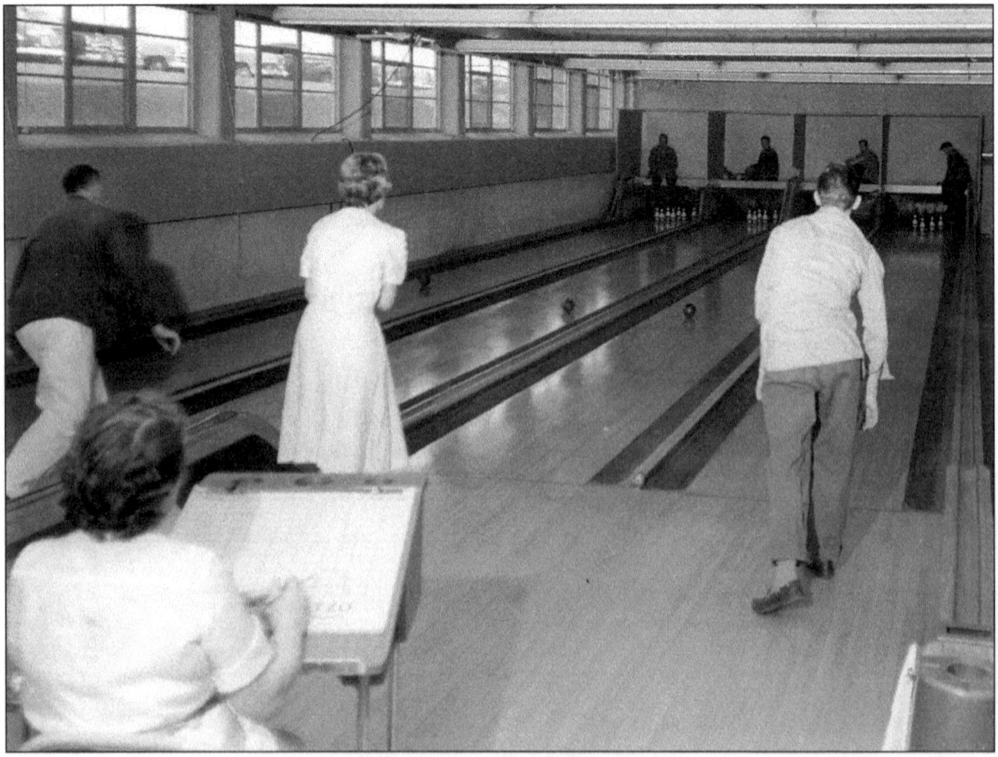

The bowling alley was a spacious, well-lighted room. Bowling games provided exercise and recreation for patients. Patient pinsetters can be seen at the rear of the bowling alley in the c. 1956 photograph above. Another large and well-lighted basement room was home to ping pong games, which were greatly enjoyed by the patients, as seen below around 1956. (Both, courtesy of Brian Girasoli.)

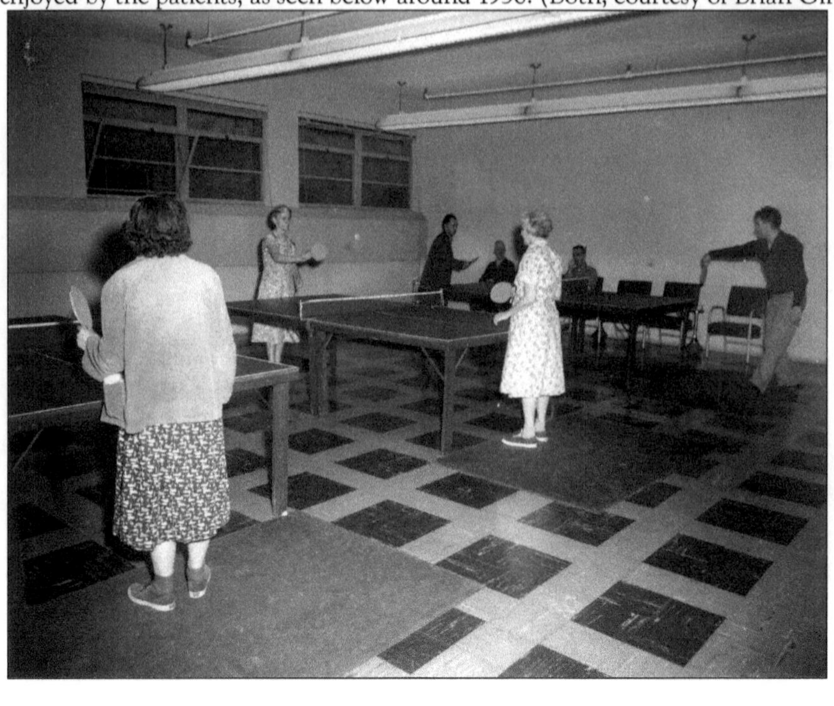

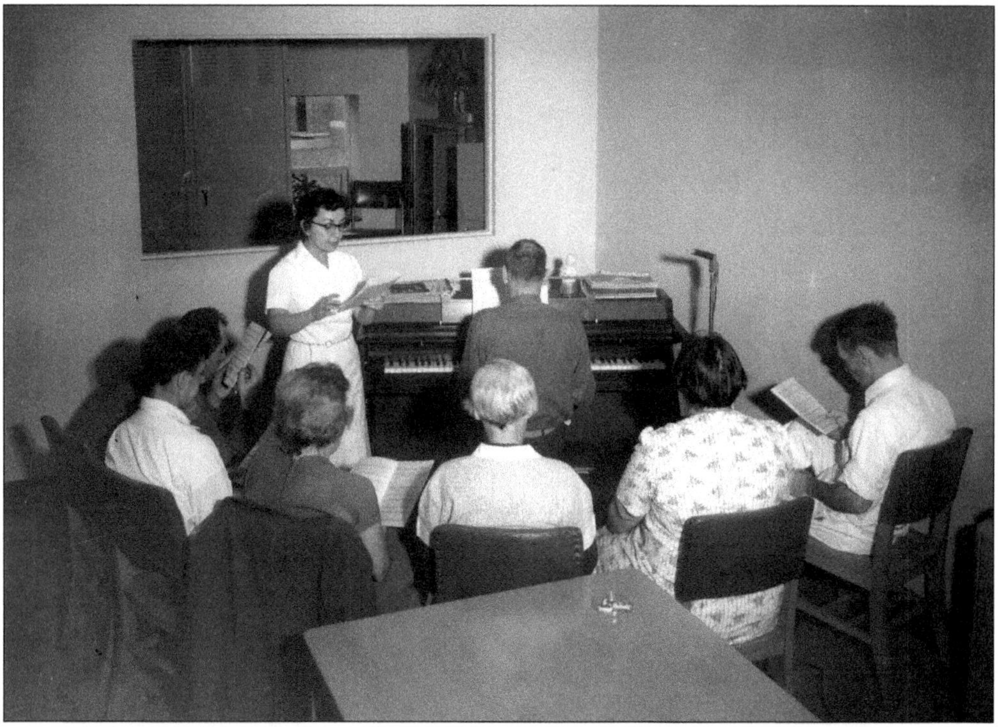

The second floor of the Russell Building was home to a radio broadcasting studio where musical programs were broadcast throughout the hospital every day. These programs were announced by the patients, who wrote their own scripts. Reviews of hospital sports activities, tape recordings of programs from commercial radio, and live programs directed by the patients were also broadcast. A live broadcast is shown above, while a staff member aids a patient in the broadcast control room below; both images were captured around 1956. (Both, courtesy of Brian Girasoli.)

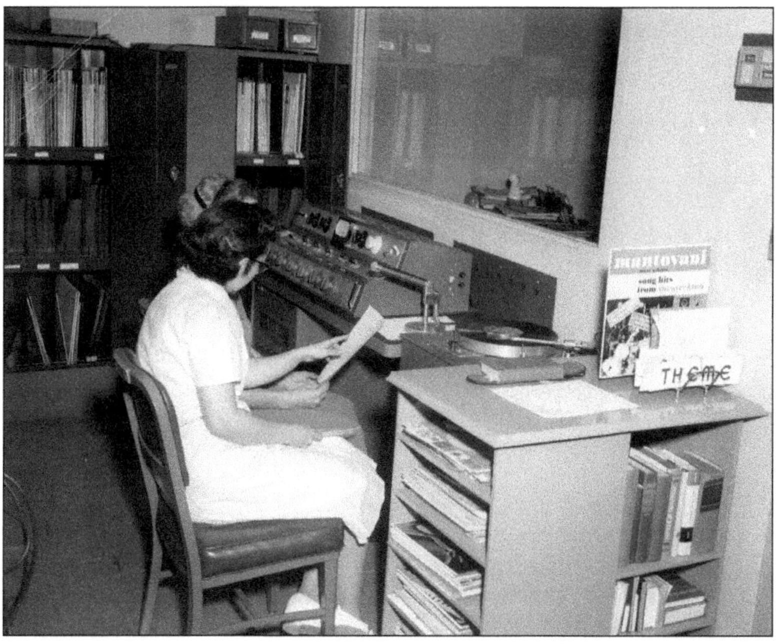

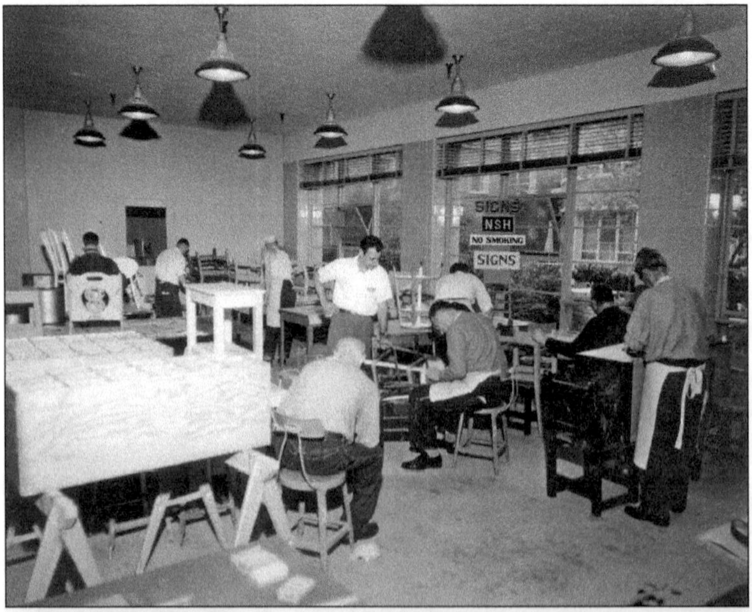

All signs used throughout NSH were made in the Russell Building's paint shop. Hospital staff directed patients on how to create the signs. The paint shop is also where wood furniture made in Russell's woodshop, such as chairs, tables, and nightstands, were painted and readied for use on the wards. (Courtesy of Brian Girasoli.)

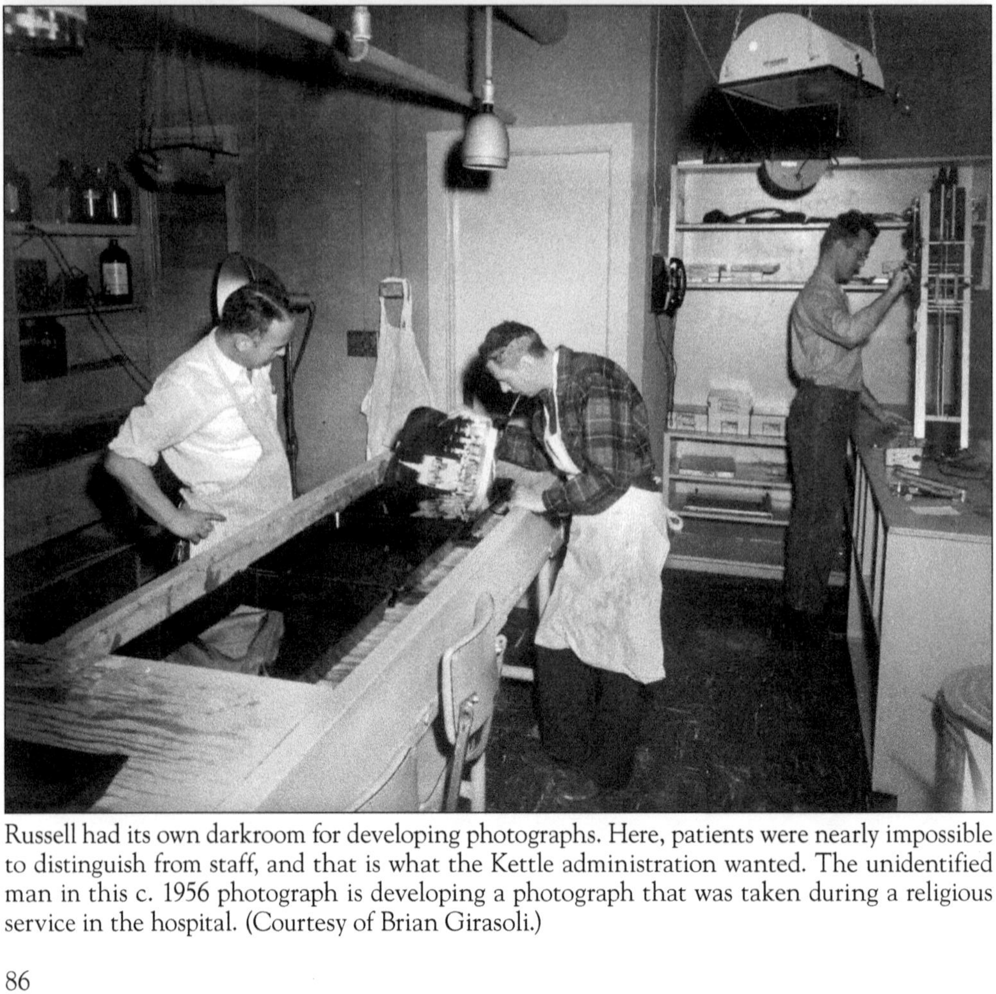

Russell had its own darkroom for developing photographs. Here, patients were nearly impossible to distinguish from staff, and that is what the Kettle administration wanted. The unidentified man in this c. 1956 photograph is developing a photograph that was taken during a religious service in the hospital. (Courtesy of Brian Girasoli.)

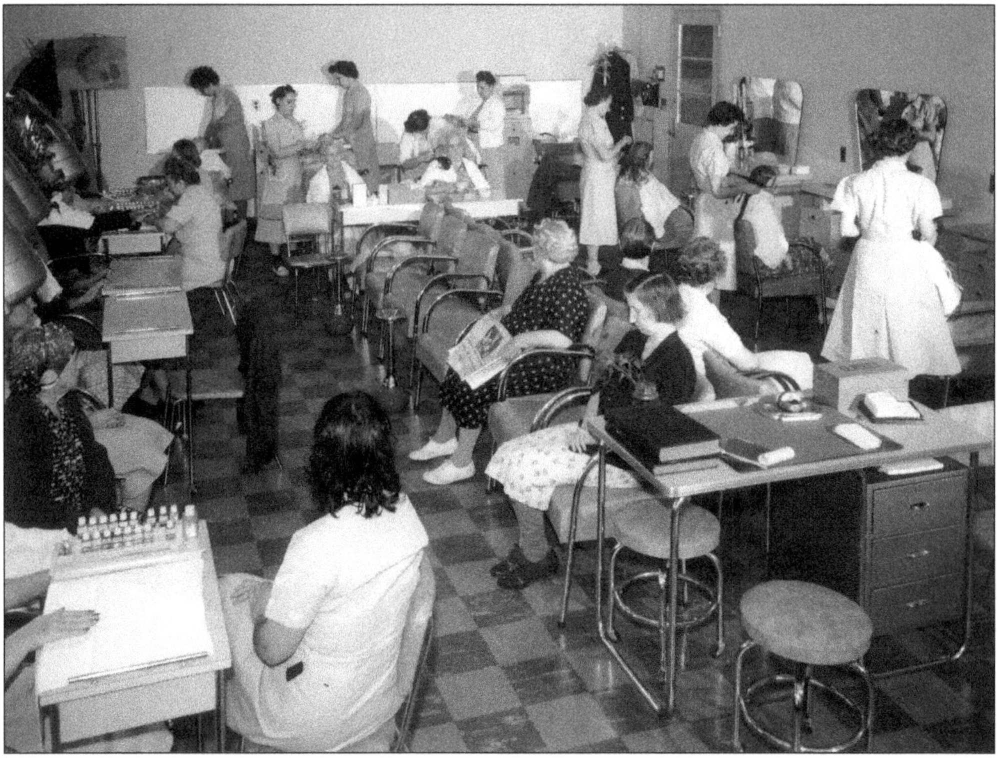

A beauty parlor for female patients (above) and a barbershop for male patients (below) were on the first floor of the Russell Building. Female patients were able to go to the beauty parlor to have their hair done in styles that pleased them, doing away with the "bug house cut" they previously wore and hated in the early 1940s. Manicures were also done to help boost female patients' self-image. Male patients frequented the barbershop to have their hair cut in any style of their choosing. (Both, courtesy of Brian Girasoli.)

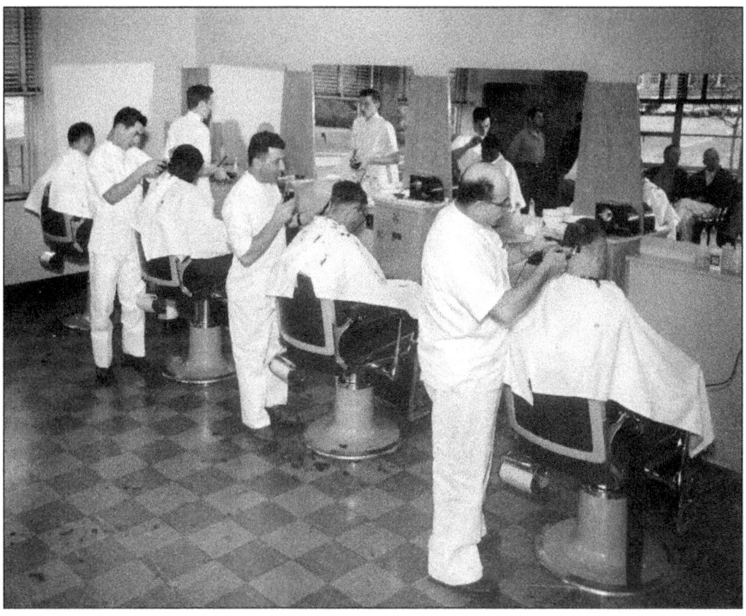

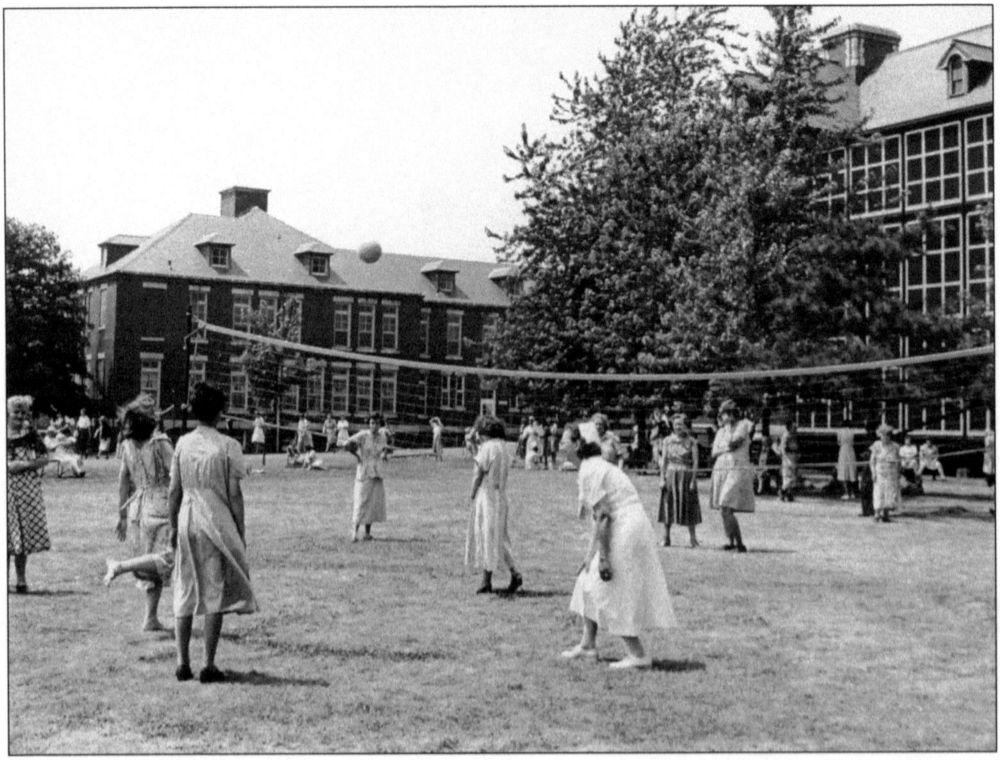

Outdoor exercise and activities such as volleyball, pictured above, were a vital part of the OT program. Patients were strongly urged not to remain in a sedentary state and to join in the fun, even if all they could physically do was watch and enjoy from the sidelines. Engaging patients in a physically active and social atmosphere was imperative to recovery from mental illness. The date of this photograph is unknown. (Courtesy of Kristen Polci-Parsons.)

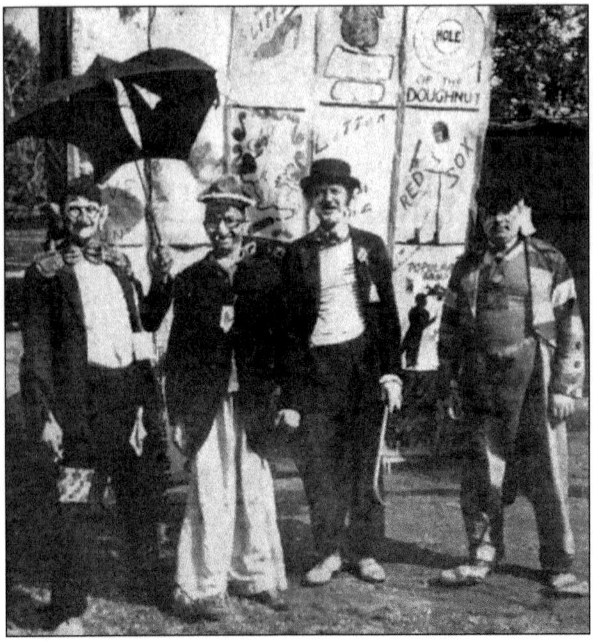

Harry Kromer and his occupational therapy department became nationally known for writing the best prescriptions for Norwich State Hospital's patients: a day of outdoor fun at the therapeutic carnival. Each fall, the local Elks Club sponsored this carnival for over 2,000 patients with streamers hung between the buildings, bingo booths, and other games where patients won prizes, took part in outdoor races, and enjoyed refreshments. NSH staff is pictured here in 1955 dressed as clowns for the carnival, which was greatly enjoyed by all. (Author's collection.)

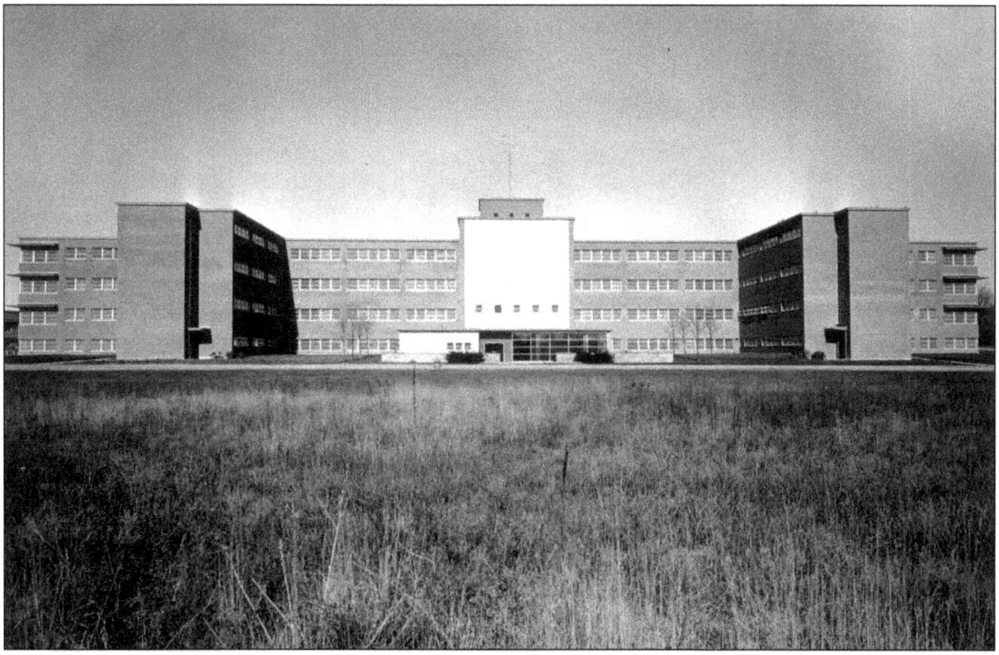

The Lodge Building was the next to rise during the expansion of the 1950s. The beautiful new four-story modern building was complete with a basement that was connected to Norwich State Hospital's massive tunnel system. The opening of Lodge, pictured above around 1956, brought the closure of the dilapidated Butler, Cutter, and Dix women's wards. Female patients from these buildings were moved to Lodge, where they initially were not receptive to their colorful, cheerful, and modern new home. Many patients threatened to destroy the building before becoming accustomed to their new surroundings. (Courtesy of Brian Girasoli.)

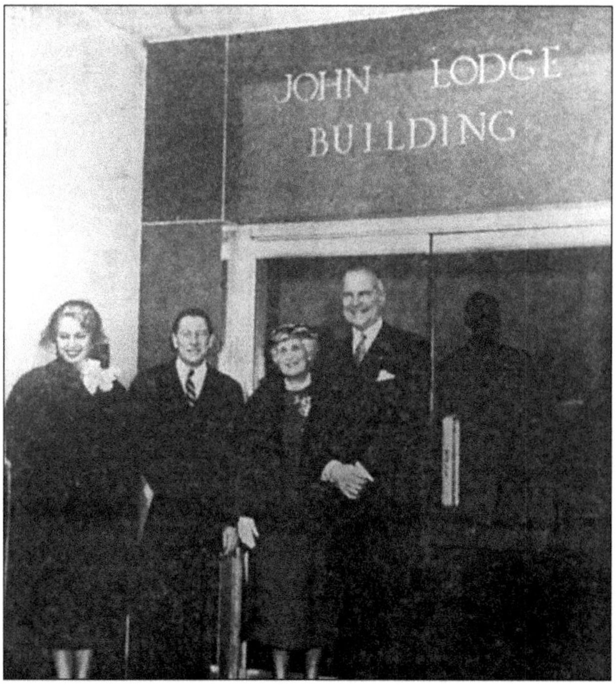

The Lodge Building was named for former Connecticut governor John Davis Lodge for his support and contributions to the fight against mental diseases. The building was opened with formal ceremonies on December 28, 1956. Governor Lodge is shown at far right standing outside the main entrance to the new building. Also pictured are, from left to right, Mrs. John D. Lodge, Philip A. Johnson (chairman of the hospital's board of trustees), and his wife. (Author's collection.)

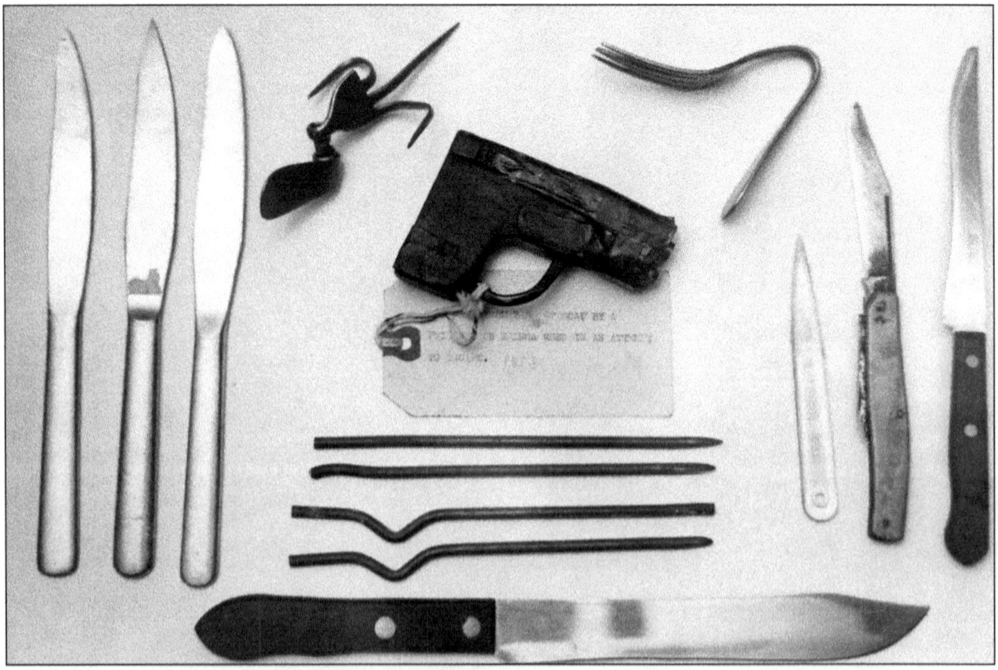

Amidst Norwich State Hospital's exciting new building growth, Dr. Kettle remained faced with one problem that continuously tried to blacken the reputation of the hospital: the inadequate Salmon Building, which housed the criminally insane. Pictured above are weapons that patients made from hospital cutlery and nails from various industrial shops. Patients would file butter knives to a fine, deadly point in their rooms. One patient made a fake gun from a bar of soap and electrical tape (above, center) in an attempt to escape in 1958. Pictured below are more items patients smuggled back to their wards from various industrial shops for escape attempts and other harmful purposes. Contraband items such as these were confiscated by hospital staff and Norwich State Hospital police. (Both, courtesy of Patti Daniels.)

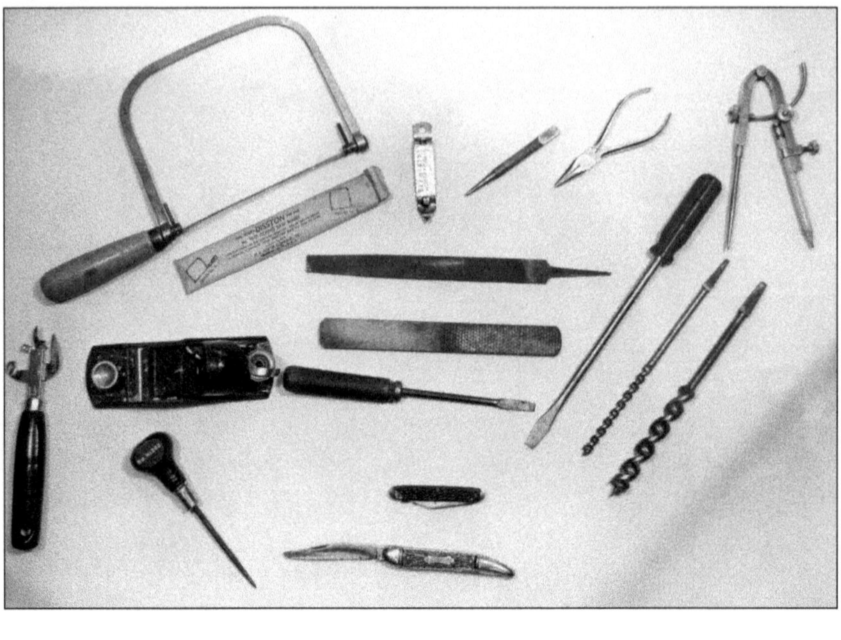

Ulysses S. Nygren was one of many patients who succeeded in escaping the Salmon Building. His escapes were detailed in local newspapers. Pictured is one of his drawings done while an inpatient at NSH, dated April 8, 1979. Repeated escapes made the community ill at ease and darkened NSH's reputation. The state refused to close Salmon and move criminally insane patients out of Norwich until 1971, when a new forensic security treatment center was opened at Connecticut Valley Hospital in Middletown. (Author's collection.)

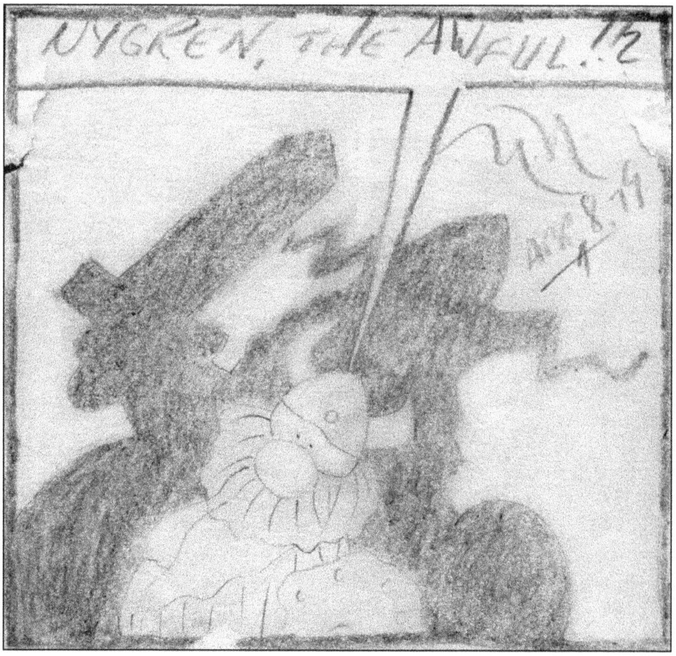
NYGREN, THE AWFUL!!2

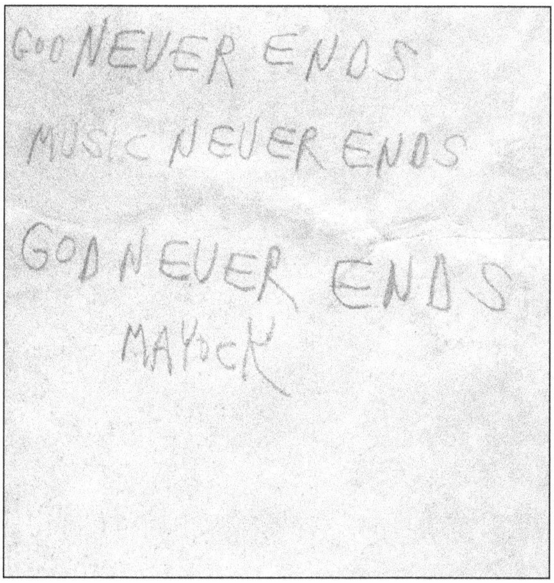
GOD NEVER ENDS
MUSIC NEVER ENDS
GOD NEVER ENDS
MAYOCK

Peter Mayock, known in local newspapers as "Prophet Peter," repeatedly appealed to the court for his release from Norwich State Hospital in the 1950s and 1960s. Mayock was committed in 1914 and again in 1917 for literally obeying the biblical injunction, "If thy right eye offend thee, pluck it out and if thy right hand offend thee, cut it off," defending his actions by stating that he had a constitutional right to his self-maiming. Pictured here is the back of a slip of paper from Otis Library in Norwich written on by Mayock while at Norwich State Hospital. He would later become an inspiration to Norwich native author Wally Lamb in his novel *I Know This Much Is True*. (Author's collection.)

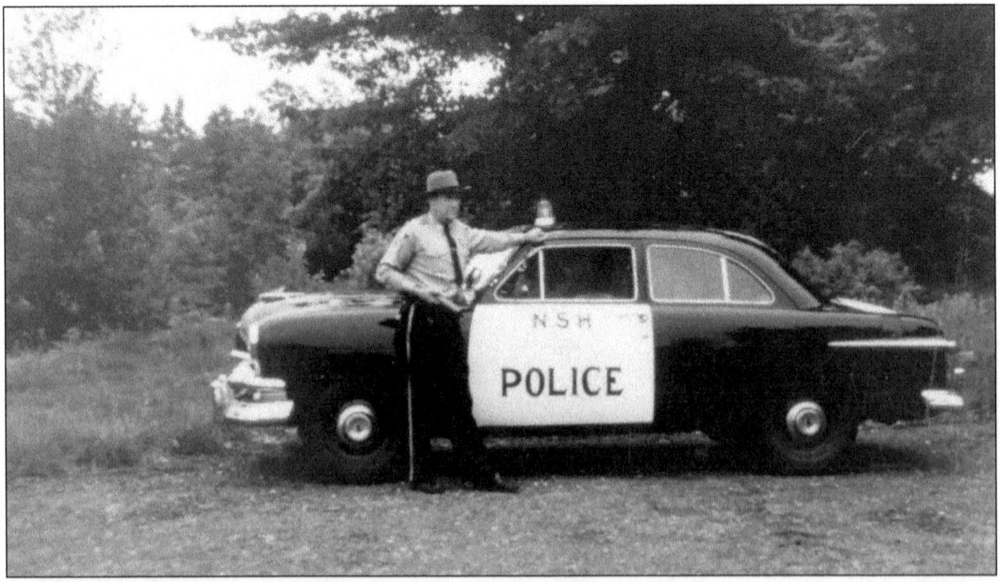

Because Norwich State Hospital and other psychiatric hospitals across the country housed dangerously ill patients like the criminally insane, Norwich State Hospital had its own police force to patrol and monitor hospital grounds. Pictured is Capt. George McGowan with his NSH patrol car around the 1950s. (Courtesy of Patti Daniels.)

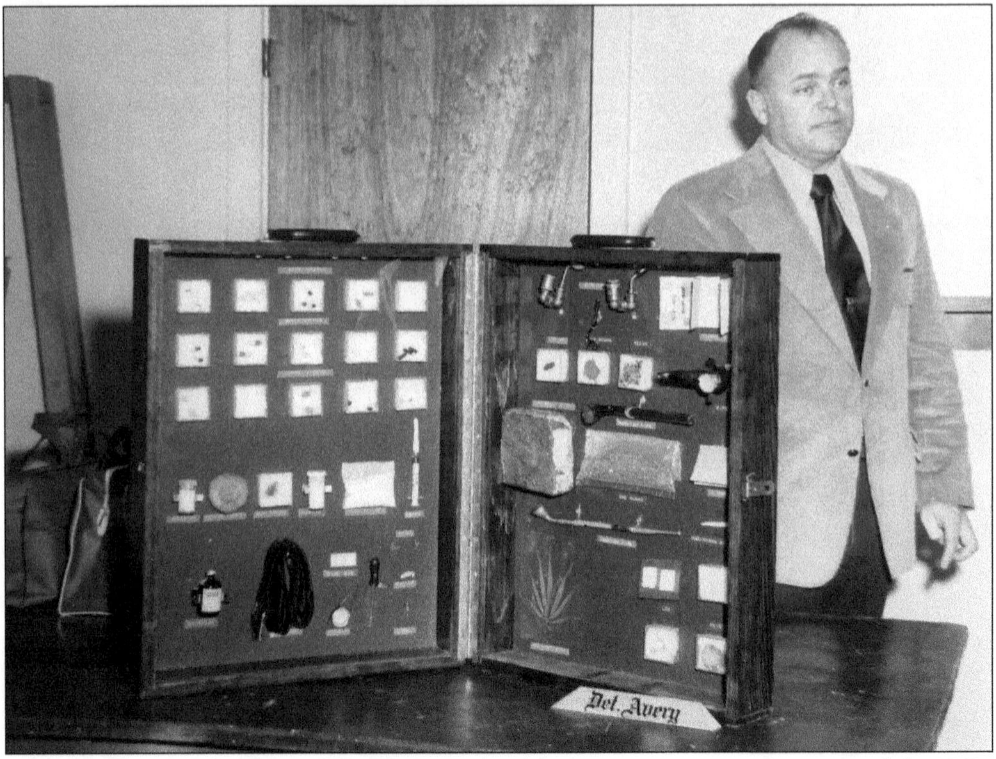

Detective Avery of the Norwich State Hospital police department is seen here around the 1960s educating staff on the various types of narcotic and illegal drug substances they might find hidden in patient's rooms and on the wards. (Courtesy of Patti Daniels.)

Norwich State Hospital police were on site to document incidents of patient outbursts that resulted in day rooms being tossed and trashed, as pictured here around the 1950s. The nurse in the photograph is unidentified. (Courtesy of Patti Daniels.)

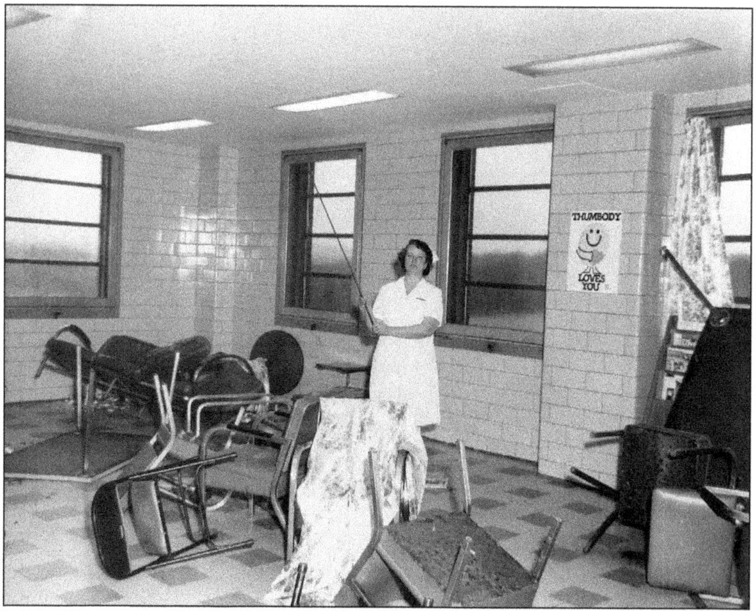

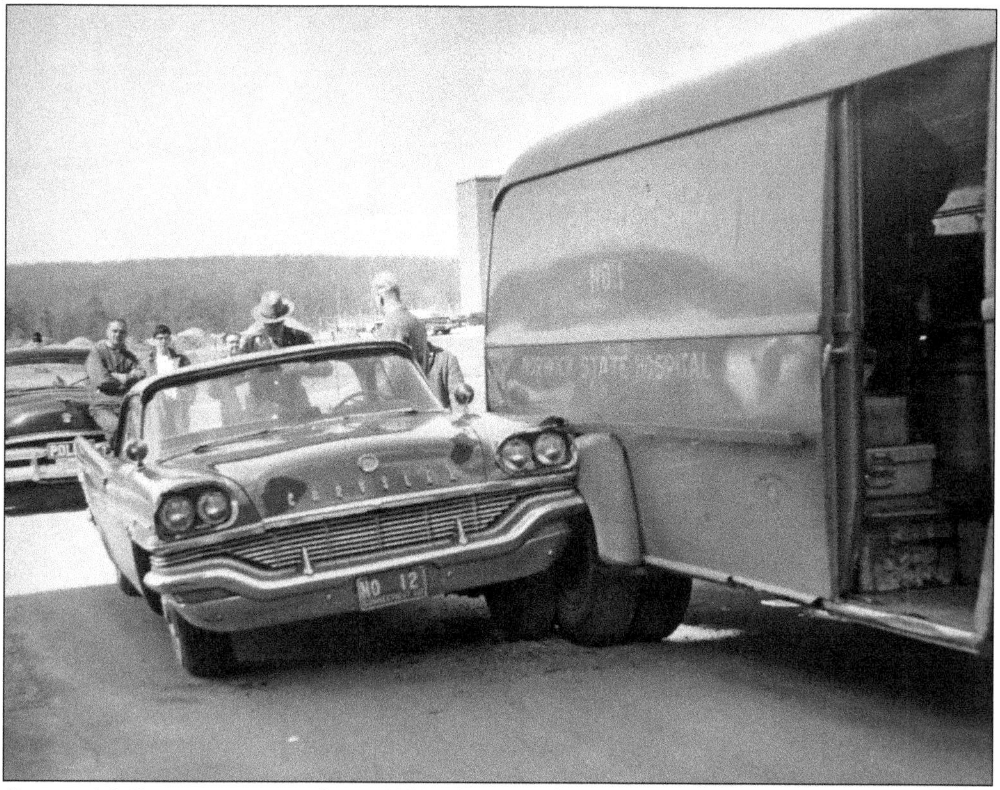

Captain McGowan is seen in this c. 1950s photograph writing a ticket for an accident involving one of Norwich State Hospital's food service trucks on Route 12. (Courtesy of Patti Daniels.)

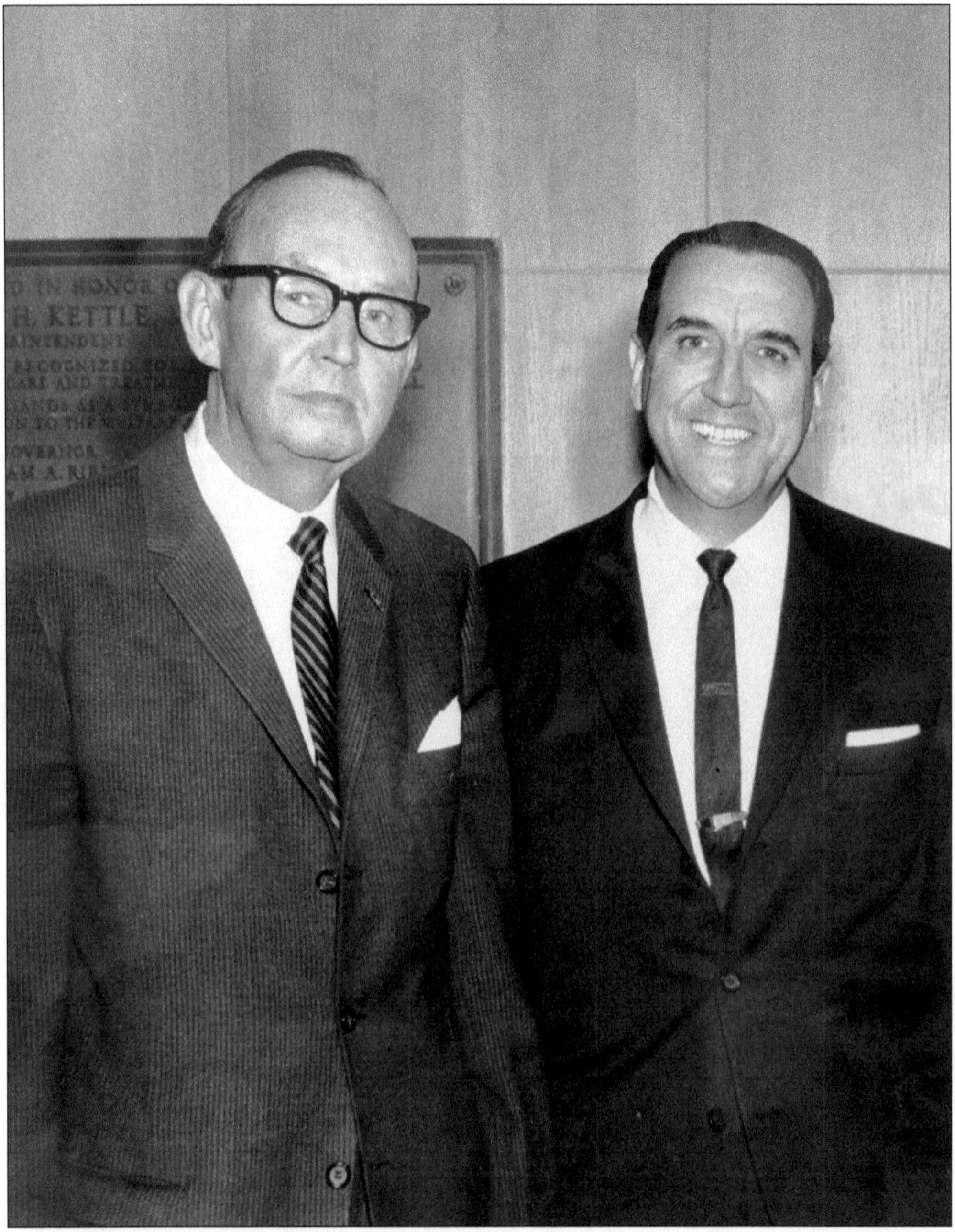

Dr. Ronald H. Kettle (left) is pictured here beside former Connecticut governor John. N. Dempsey, around 1961. Governor Dempsey lauded Dr. Kettle for all his innovative efforts that updated and brought Norwich State Hospital into the era of modern psychiatric patient care. One more important task had to be done to complete Norwich State Hospital's new modern image: the unpleasant connotation of the word "state" in the hospital's name needed to finally be eliminated. Former Connecticut governor Abraham Ribicoff, whom Governor Dempsey succeeded, was instrumental in enabling the General Assembly to pass the legislation enacting the name change. On October 1, 1961, Norwich State Hospital's name changed for a third and final time to Norwich Hospital. (Courtesy of Patti Daniels.)

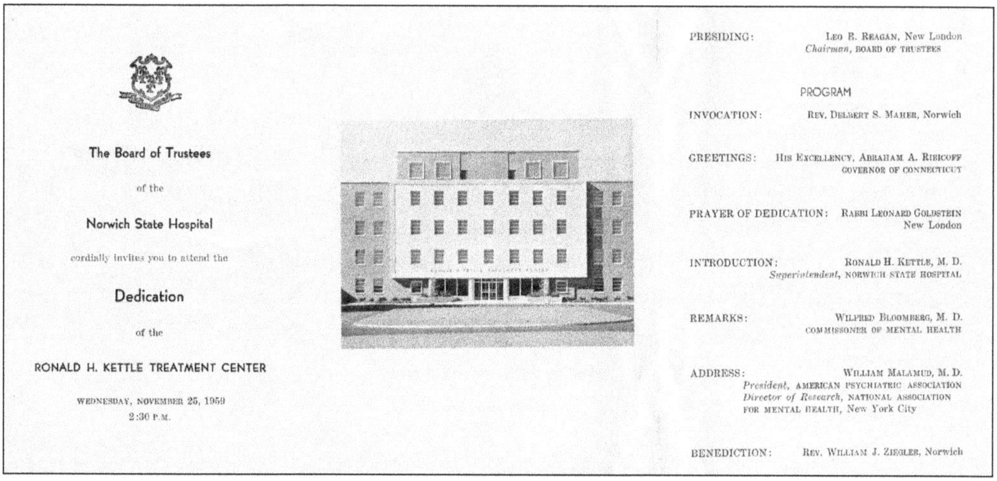

The Board of Trustees

of the

Norwich State Hospital

cordially invites you to attend the

Dedication

of the

RONALD H. KETTLE TREATMENT CENTER

WEDNESDAY, NOVEMBER 25, 1959
2:30 P.M.

PRESIDING: LEO B. REAGAN, New London
Chairman, BOARD OF TRUSTEES

PROGRAM

INVOCATION: REV. DELBERT S. MAHER, Norwich

GREETINGS: HIS EXCELLENCY, ABRAHAM A. RIBICOFF
GOVERNOR OF CONNECTICUT

PRAYER OF DEDICATION: RABBI LEONARD GOLDSTEIN
New London

INTRODUCTION: RONALD H. KETTLE, M. D.
Superintendent, NORWICH STATE HOSPITAL

REMARKS: WILFRED BLOOMBERG, M. D.
COMMISSONER OF MENTAL HEALTH

ADDRESS: WILLIAM MALAMUD, M. D.
President, AMERICAN PSYCHIATRIC ASSOCIATION
Director of Research, NATIONAL ASSOCIATION FOR MENTAL HEALTH, New York City

BENEDICTION: REV. WILLIAM J. ZIEGLER, Norwich

The largest building on the campus, the Ronald H. Kettle Treatment Center, opened with official ceremonies on November 25, 1959. Pictured above is an official invitation to the formal opening of the new center, showing the building's façade. These invitations were distributed to dignitaries and interested parties. The new Kettle Treatment Center was a massive brick four-story modern hospital building complete with a basement that connected to all the other buildings via Norwich Hospital's tunnel system. The Kettle Building was designed as an admission and intensive treatment unit with 12 wards for both sexes. Brand new state-of-the-art X-ray facilities, along with departments for dentistry, nursing education, psychology, and social services were also located in this building. A large medical library, classrooms, conference rooms, and a large auditorium were also housed here. For the first time in Norwich Hospital's history, all these departments were centralized and organized under one roof. (Author's collection.)

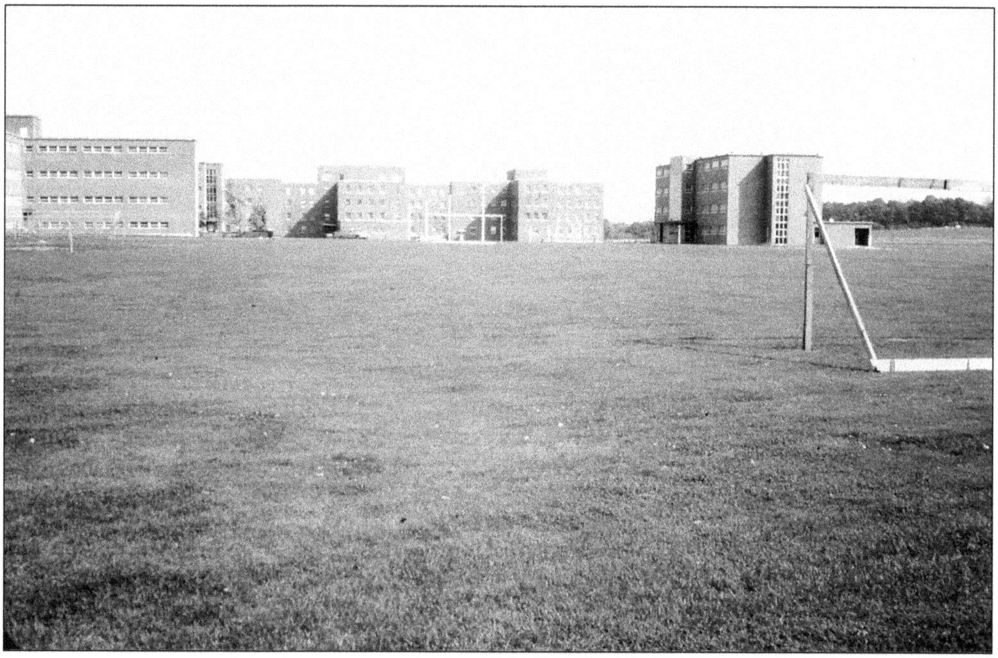

From the hospital's playing field in 1964, the rear of the Kettle Building can be seen in the distant center with a portion of Lodge to the left and the Abraham Ribicoff Research Center standing alone on the right. (Courtesy of Allan Burns.)

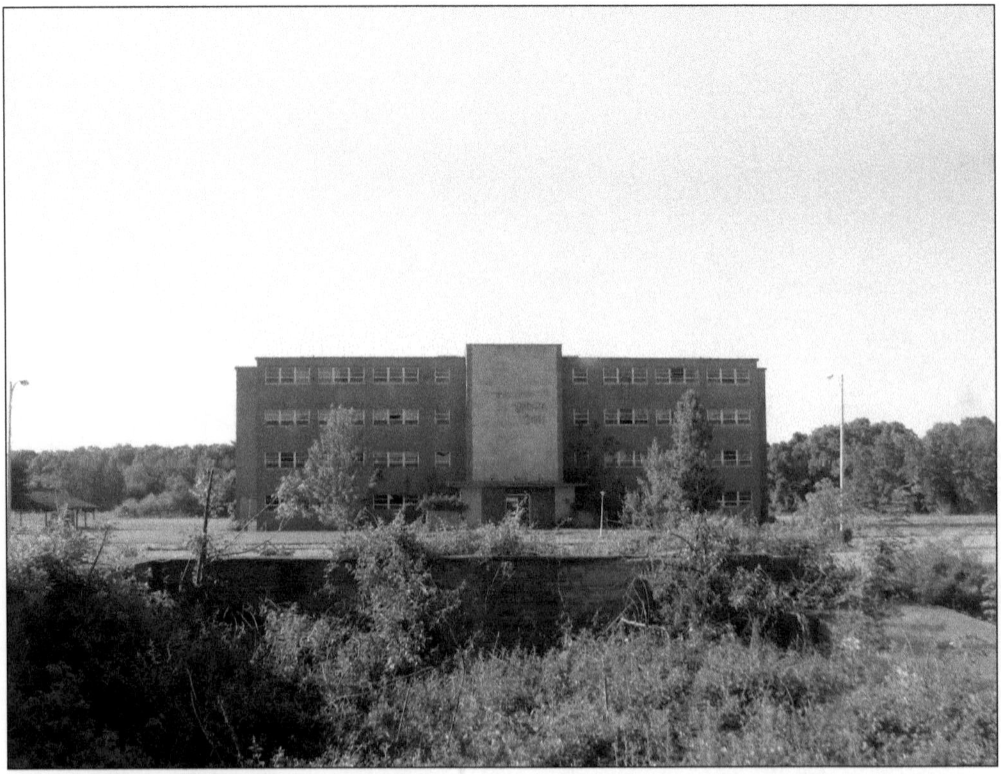

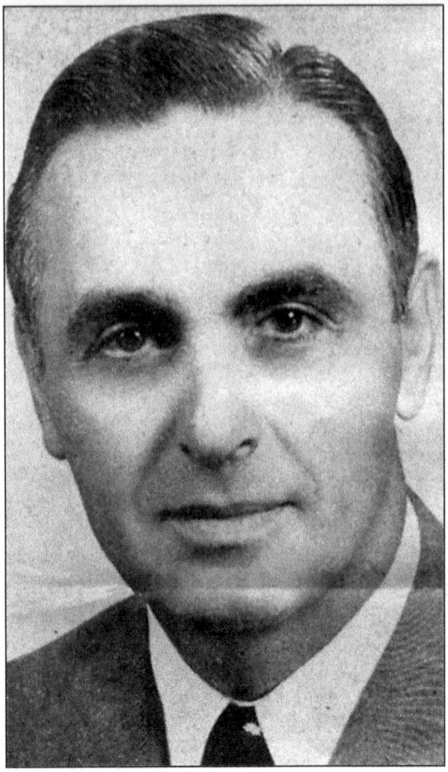

The next building to be erected during Norwich Hospital's expansion boom was the Abraham Ribicoff Research Center, pictured here in its abandoned state 14 years after NSH closed. The building was created for mental health research in hopes of better understanding the causes of mental illness and aiding in developing pharmaceuticals to benefit sufferers. The opening of this research laboratory on NSH grounds enabled the hospital to transfer all its laboratory activities from its tiny, old building to this beautiful new four-story modern building. The Abraham Ribicoff Research Center contained histology, neuropathology, and biochemistry labs, along with doctors' offices, conference rooms, classrooms, operating rooms for testing on animals, and a morgue. The work done in this laboratory benefited all three of Connecticut's state hospitals. (Author's collection.)

The research center was named for former Connecticut governor Abraham A. Ribicoff, seen here, for his staunch support of Norwich Hospital administration and the work done in helping those afflicted with mental illness. The research center was formally opened on November 8, 1962. (Author's collection.)

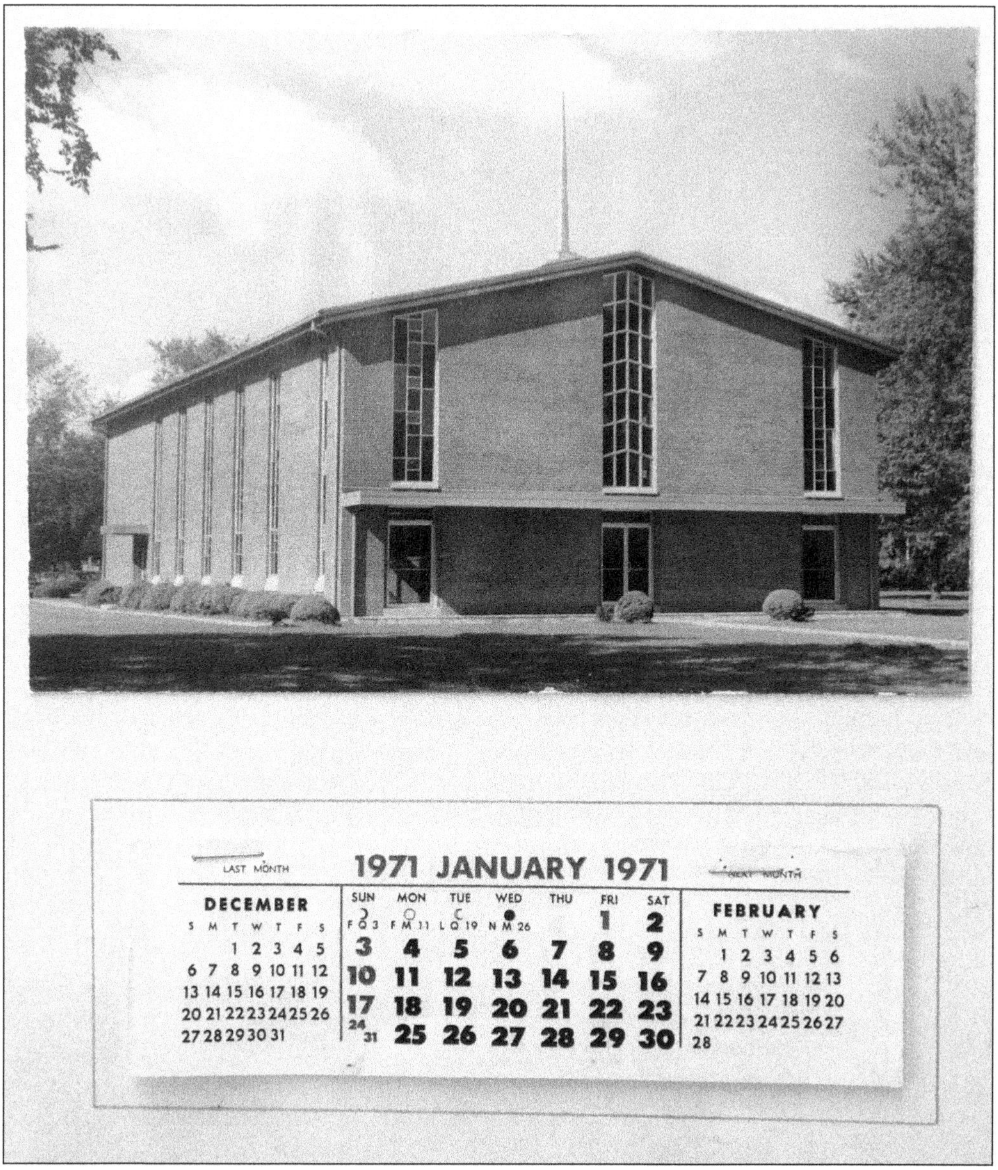

The final addition to the Norwich Hospital campus was an interdenominational chapel, pictured here. The chapel sat in front of the Administration Building and along Route 12 and was clearly visible to traffic. The chapel originated from a special chapel committee appointed by Governor Ribicoff in 1955 to recognize "that spiritual as well as the physical welfare of those under the state's care is of great importance." Governor Dempsey spoke these words during the dedication ceremony for the interdenominational chapel on March 15, 1962. Norwich Hospital was the second institution in Connecticut to have an interfaith chapel. The chapel was designed to accommodate religious services for Catholic, Protestant, and Jewish faiths. Approximately 600 people could be seated very comfortably in the attractive new structure. Many Norwich Hospital employee couples were married here. (Courtesy of Patti Daniels.)

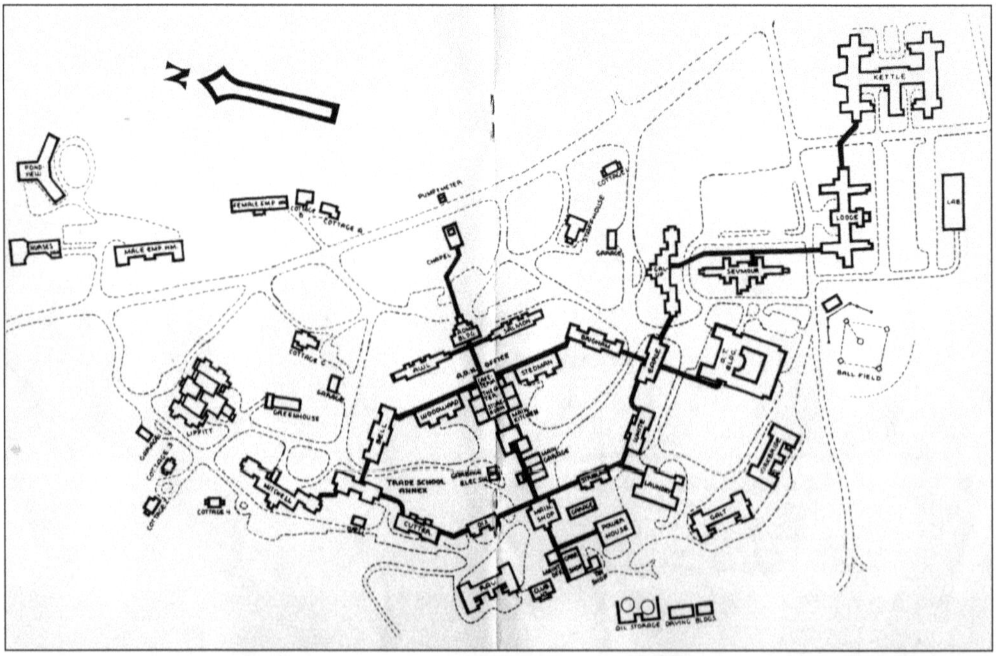

The map above, from after 1962, shows the completed arrangement of Norwich Hospital's ward buildings, complex tunnel system, staff housing, and physician's cottages. The Bryan Building and the physicians' homes on Hospital Hill are not pictured. By 1970, the entire hospital property spanned both the city of Norwich and the town of Preston and was over 900 acres in size with over 75 buildings. By the 1980s, most of the original ward buildings were closed. Cutter, Dix, and White were demolished by the mid-1970s. Their removal, especially White, was highly significant to the new era of patient care Norwich Hospital was dedicated to providing. A small ceremony among hospital employees was held marking the bygone darker days. As each brick fell from White, employees rejoiced, knowing that the days of bare patients living in feces and squalor were nothing but a bad memory. White's basement, shown below in 1987, remained so that the tunnel system would not be disrupted. (Both, author's collection.)

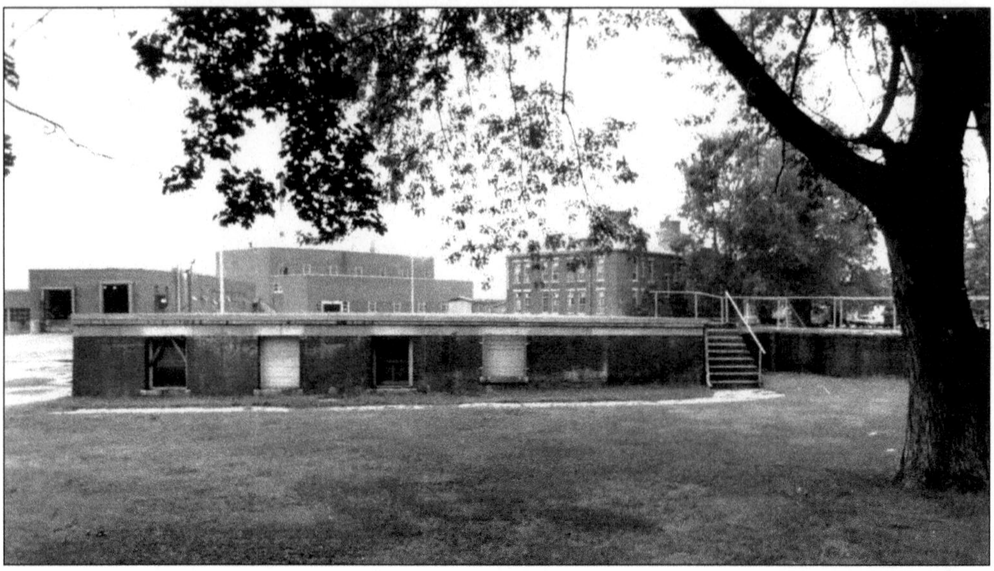

Five

The People of Norwich State Hospital

Throughout its last 35 years of operation, Norwich Hospital was well-known and well-respected in southeastern Connecticut as more than just another one of the state's three psychiatric hospitals. The selfless care and undying compassion the staff displayed for their patients and the close camaraderie that formed between employees of all departments made what was locally known as "the Shining City on the Thames" a true family. The staff never saw their work at NH as a job; NH was their lives. Norwich Hospital was one of the largest employers in southeastern Connecticut, with over 3,000 dedicated staff at its peak. Multiple generations of families passed their love of working at Norwich Hospital down to their future generations, who also treasured their work.

Norwich Hospital was threatened with closure twice: first in 1981 and again in 1992 as part of a proposed cost-saving benefit to the state budget. Former Connecticut governor John Rowland, who served one year in federal prison for using the governor's office to subvert the political process and profit personally, had signed off on contracts worth millions of dollars for improvements to NH, including an HVAC renovation and a new roof for the Kettle Building. With the work well underway, NH superintendent Garrell Mullaney was blind-sided when he received the news that the governor had announced the closure of Norwich Hospital and its sister facility, Fairfield Hills Hospital.

Norwich Hospital's closure was a travesty to both hospital employees and members of the community. Public outrage flooded local newspapers, television, and radio shows with cries from concerned citizens. Norwich employees were given very little time to find facilities, programs, and placement for patients who required long-term care. Some patients found placement, but many became homeless. Some were fortunate to be taken into NH employees' homes.

The demolition of Norwich Hospital's buildings is not reminiscent of the closeness and the bond that former employees and their families still hold today. The lifelong friendships and family bonds that were formed in those buildings are still alive today, as the history and memories of Norwich Hospital always will be.

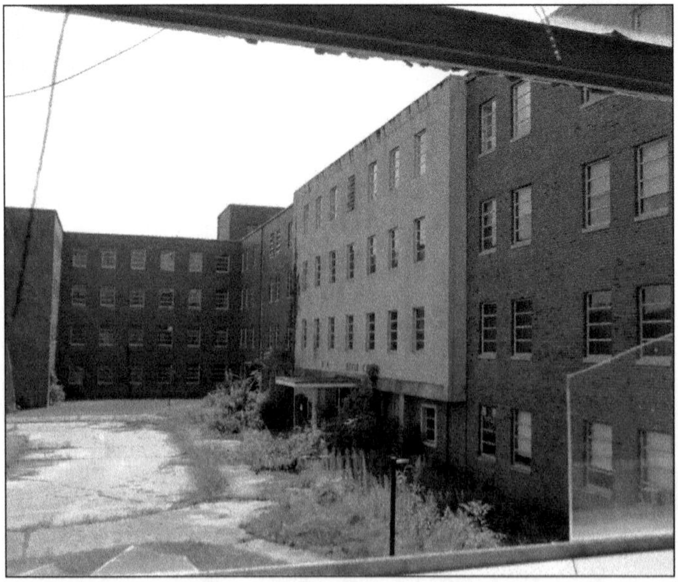

On Thursday, October 10, 1996, Norwich Hospital closed its doors forever, ending an era of 92 years of care and service to mentally ill individuals. Pictured is the Ronald H. Kettle Treatment Center in 2010 in a sad state of abandon and disrepair. The physical state of the building was comparable to the feelings of many patients who called Norwich Hospital home; abandoned without purpose, discarded without care, and left to fend for themselves. (Author's collection.)

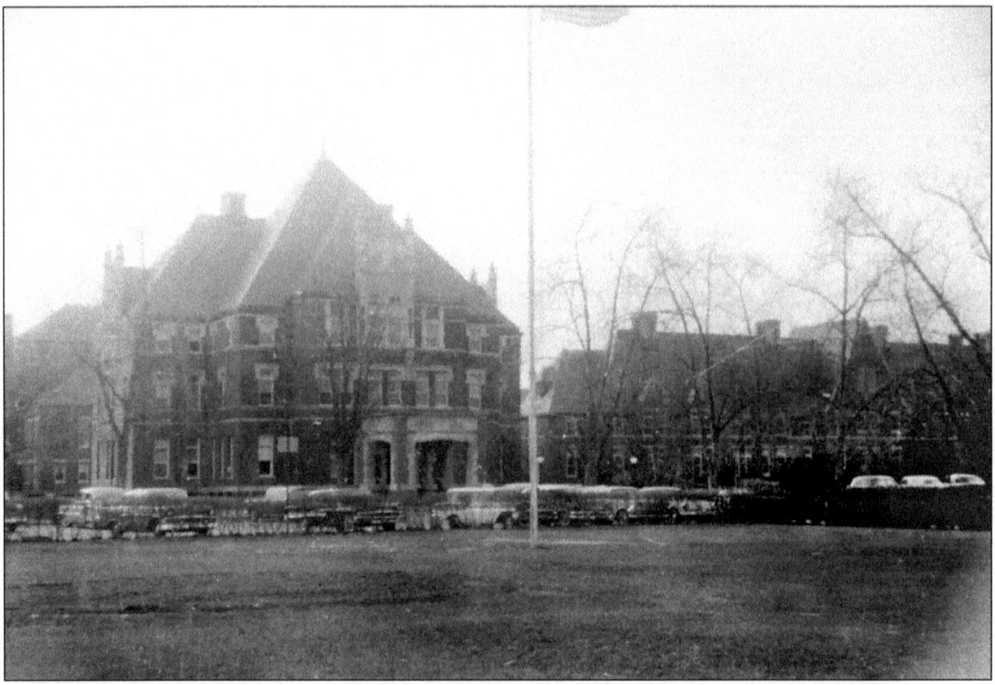

Not a single employee at the time this c. 1950 photograph of the Administration Building was taken could have imagined that their workplace, where they strived to care and remedy those with mental illness, would ever close. From the advancements of psychotropic drugs and occupational therapy programs in the 1950s, Norwich Hospital went on in future decades to experiment with various innovative programs and incentives to help its patients recover and return to their lives in society. Norwich Hospital had been built to grow with the times and always be there as a safety net for those who needed it. (Courtesy of Lloyd Langhammer.)

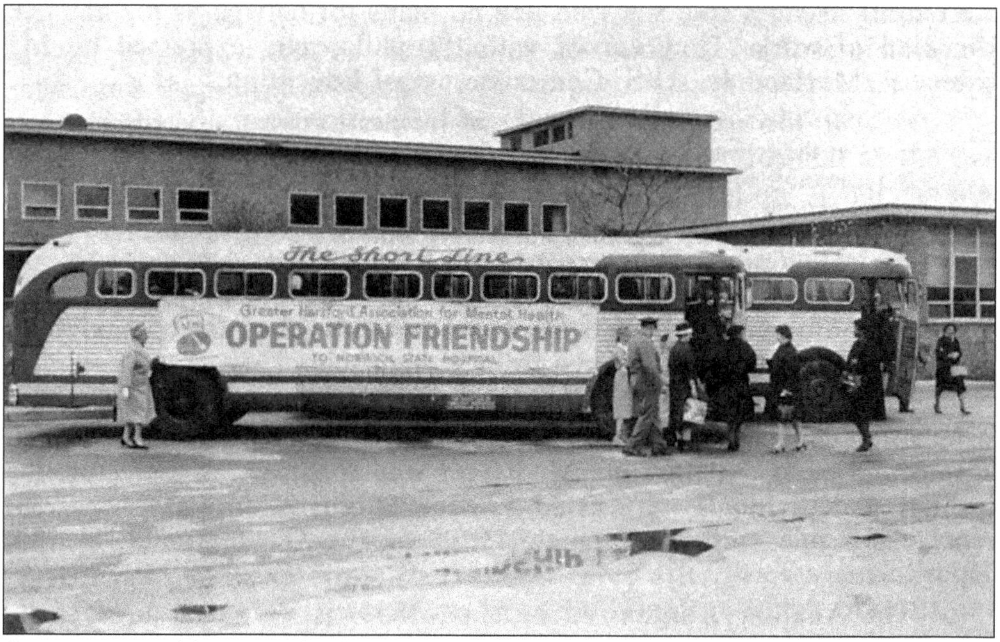

Operation Friendship was a free bus service from Hartford to Norwich Hospital provided by the Mental Health Association for families and friends of hospitalized patients. The buses, known as Sunshine Buses, operated every Sunday afternoon. A pair of Sunshine Buses is seen here parked outside the Russell Occupational Therapy Building in 1960. Dr. Kettle and his administration were proud of this endeavor. Frequent visits to the hospital from family helped to keep patients' morale up and improved their well-being. (Author's collection.)

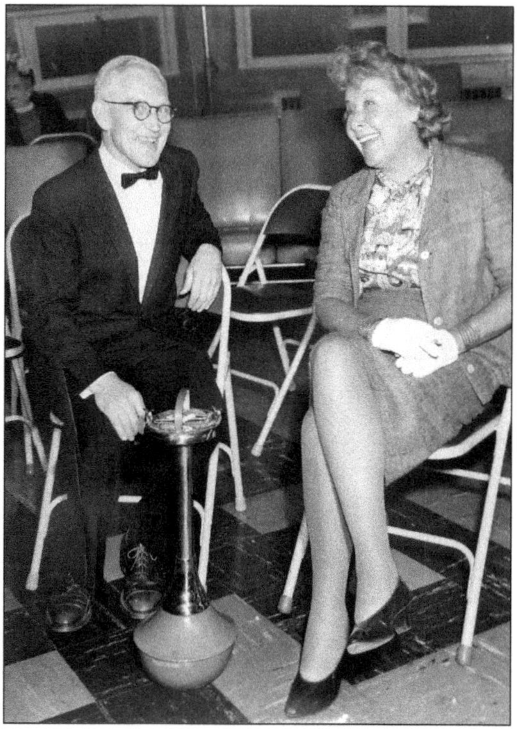

Assistant superintendent Warren Burns (left) is seated with former *I Love Lucy* star Vivian Vance in this 1964 photograph. During her tour of NSH, Vance, most remembered for her role as Ethel Mertz, sidekick to Lucille Ball, spoke of her own mental breakdown in 1954, resonating on a personal level with nearly 200 patients. (Courtesy of Allan Burns.)

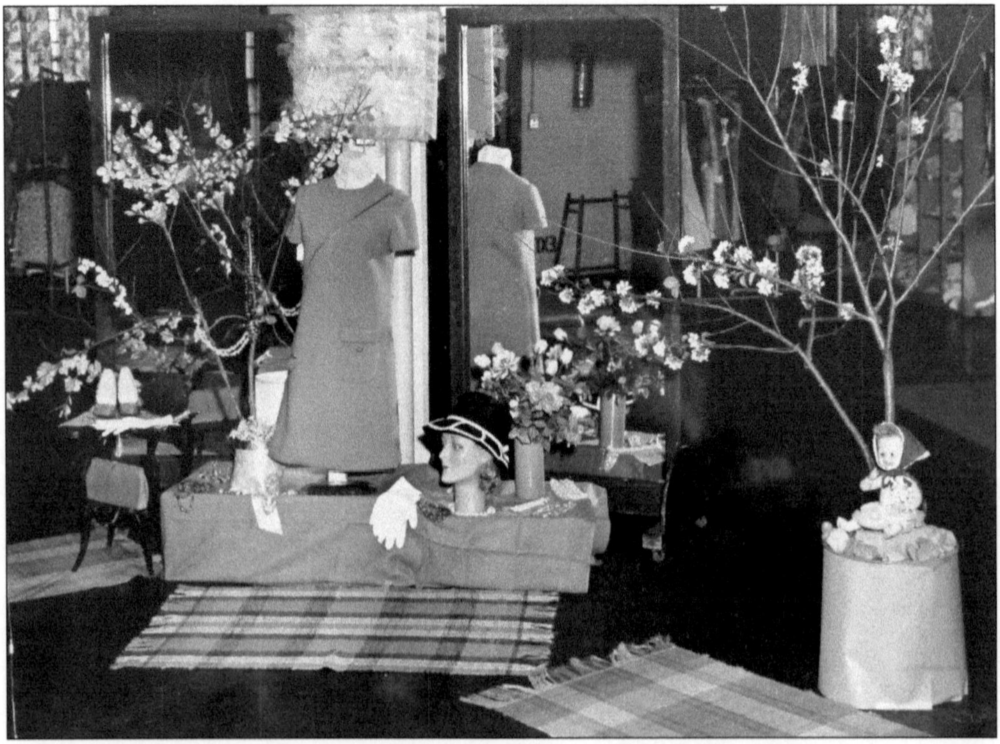

In the summer of 1961, a store for patients called the Friendly Clothing Nook was opened in the Kettle Building. Up until this time, many patients had only ill-fitting, drab state clothing that was easily identifiable as "state hospital clothing." The opening of the Friendly Clothing Nook was aimed at boosting patients' self-confidence by letting them choose and wear clothing according to their own preferences. Over 15,000 articles of clothing were donated to the beautiful store from people in the community. It was staffed by one paid employee, and hospital volunteers assisted patients in making their choices. (Both, courtesy of Kristen Polci-Parsons.)

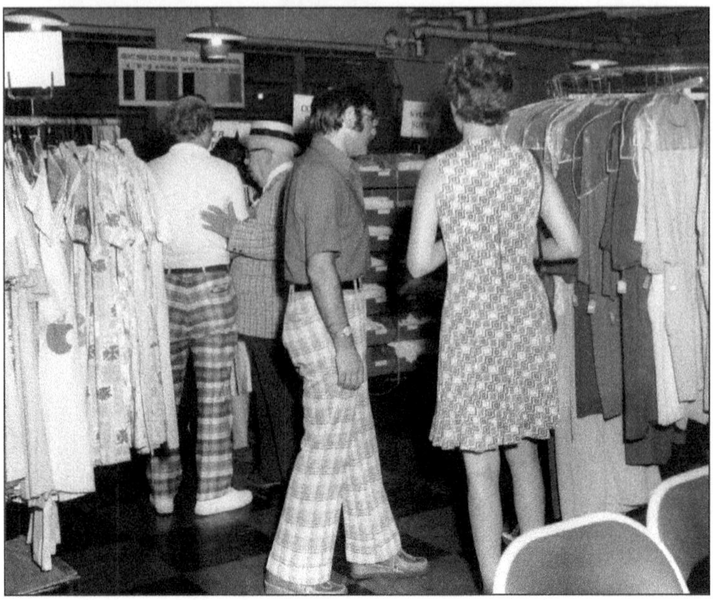

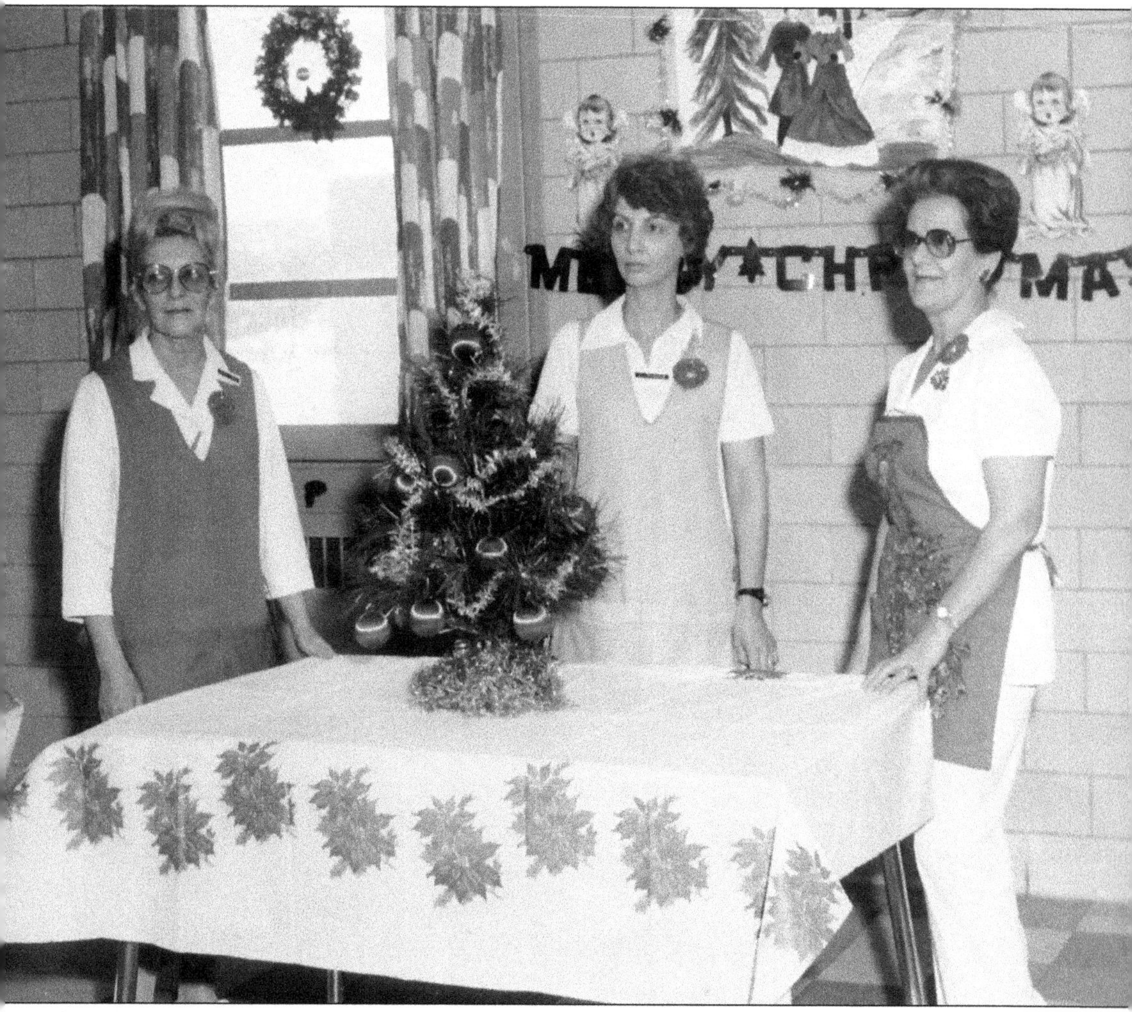

Christmas continued to be a very lively and highly celebrated time of year at Norwich Hospital. From left to right in this c. 1970 photograph, Mary Horn, Jana Laudone, and Ida DeLamentina pose in one of the wards in the Lodge Building. Norwich Hospital staff went to great lengths each year to decorate the wards and make them as happy for their patients as possible. Ward decorating contests were held each year in which the patients and staff joyously worked together to decorate their ward for the holiday season. Small prizes were given to the patients on the winning wards. (Courtesy of Kristen Polci-Parsons.)

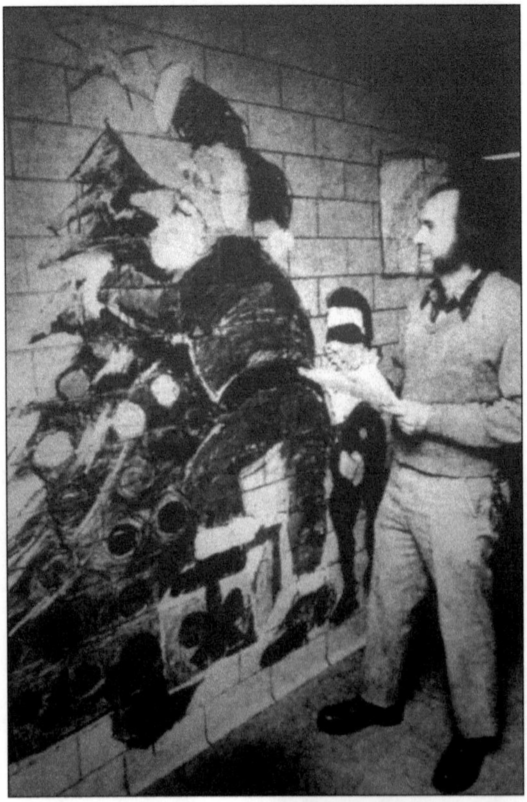

Peter Leibert judges a holiday mural painted by a patient on one of the ward walls in the Lodge Building in 1981. (Author's collection.)

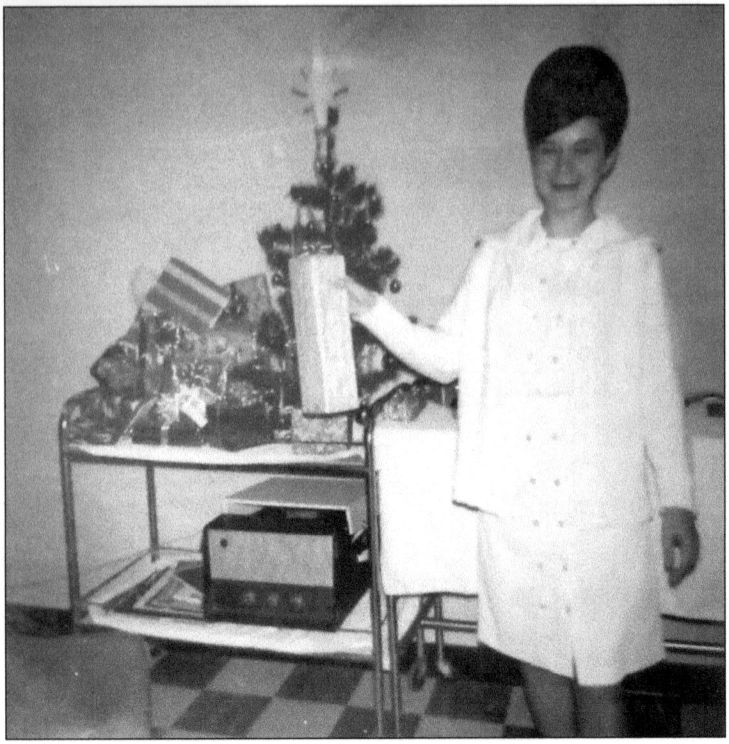

Holiday parties for Norwich Hospital staff members were held in every building. Sandra Mecienny is pictured holding a gift from a fellow worker inside the Ribicoff Research Center in 1966. (Courtesy of Ann MacDonald.)

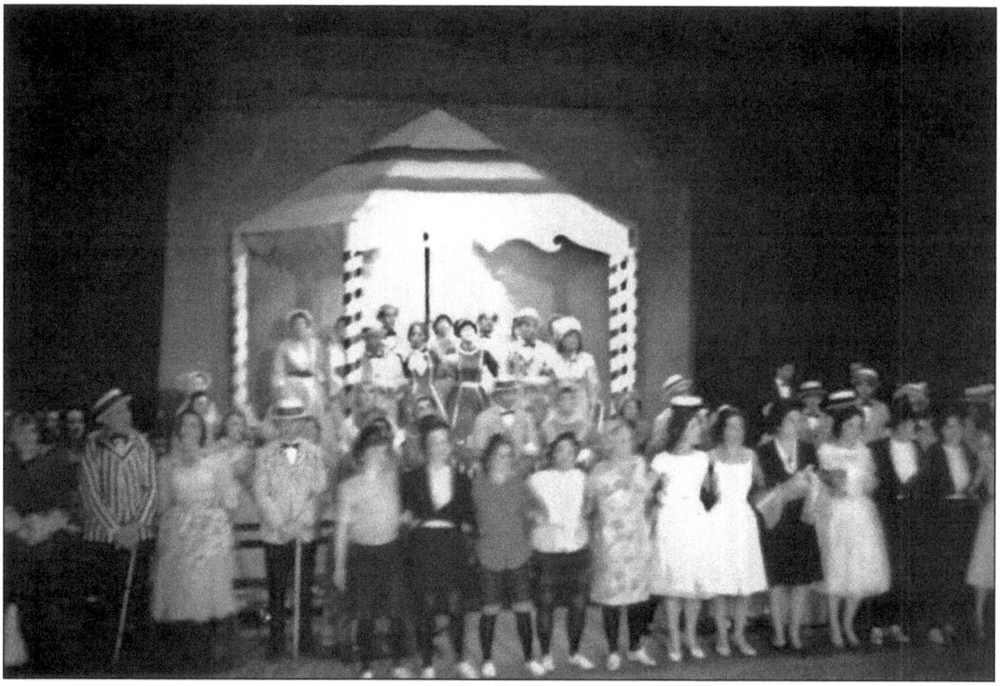

Abundant theatrical productions were put on as fundraisers and entertainment at Norwich Hospital. Both staff and patients would write, produce, and perform skits and plays. Pictured above is the NSH Freudian Follies in 1965 on the stage of the grand theater in the amusement building. On the left, the man in the striped coat and hat holding a cane and the woman in the yellow dress beside him are Norwich Hospital historian Steve DePolito's parents, Nick DePolito and Ruth DePolito. The Psychiatric Aide Association, below, also performed follies skits for entertainment in the grand theater. (Above, courtesy of Allan Burns; below, author's collection.)

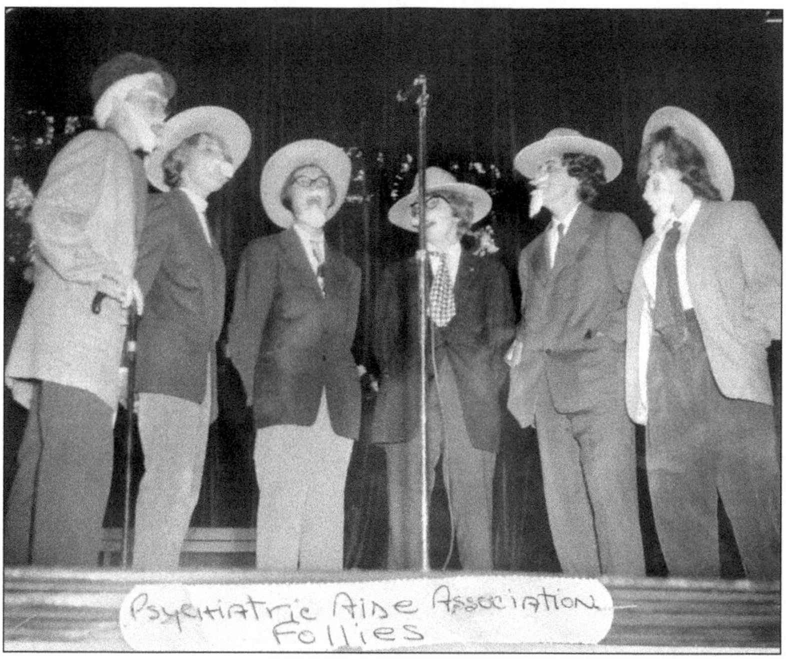

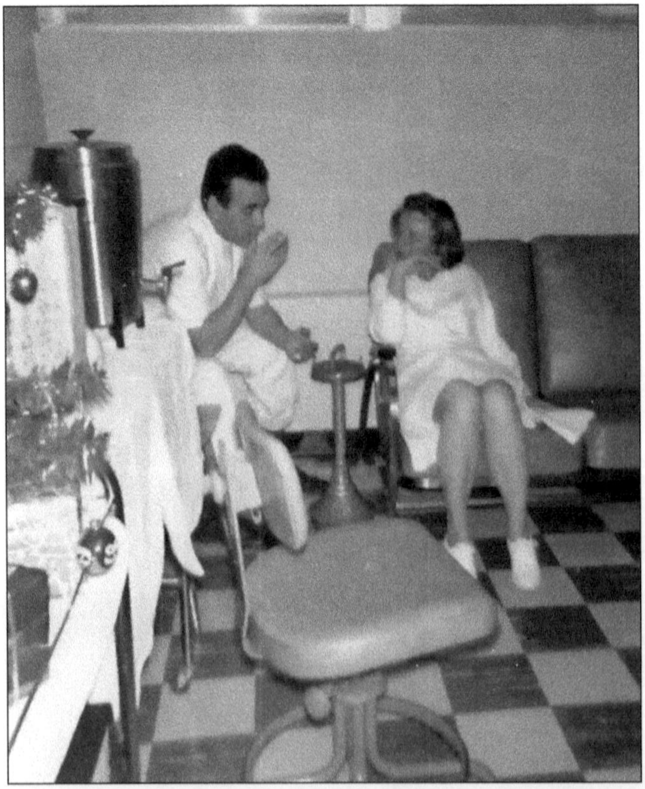

Ann MacDonald is seen here sitting next to Ralph Hartnett during the 1966 employee Christmas party inside the Ribicoff Research Center. During an interview, she recalled tales of the good-hearted "initiation rite" that new NH employees were put up to by their coworkers during their first days of work. A newcomer would be "locked" in the morgue for a very short time in the old laboratory building at the rear of the property. The joke was to offend new employees with the laboratory odors and scare them with the groaning exhales deceased bodies made when rigor mortis ceased. Ann also recalled silly pranks pulled on coworkers with an educational human skeleton in Ribicoff's morgue. (Courtesy of Ann MacDonald.)

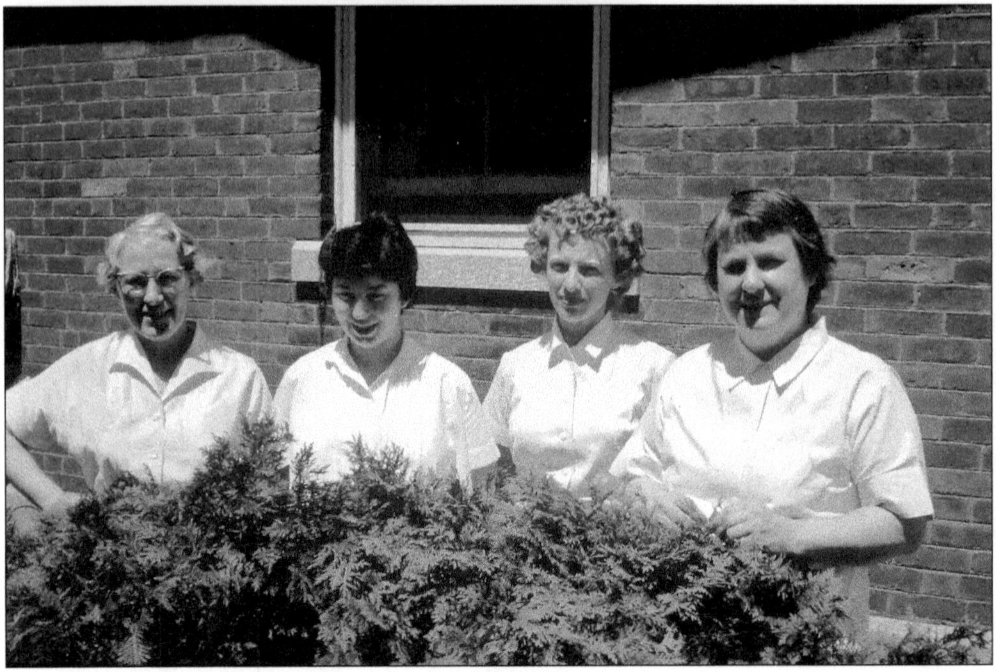

Ann MacDonald and her coworkers are pictured here in 1966, over 20 years after their portrait outside the old laboratory building taken in the 1940s. From left to right are Mary Risch, Vivian Staubley, MacDonald, and Medora Mitten. (Courtesy of Allan Burns.)

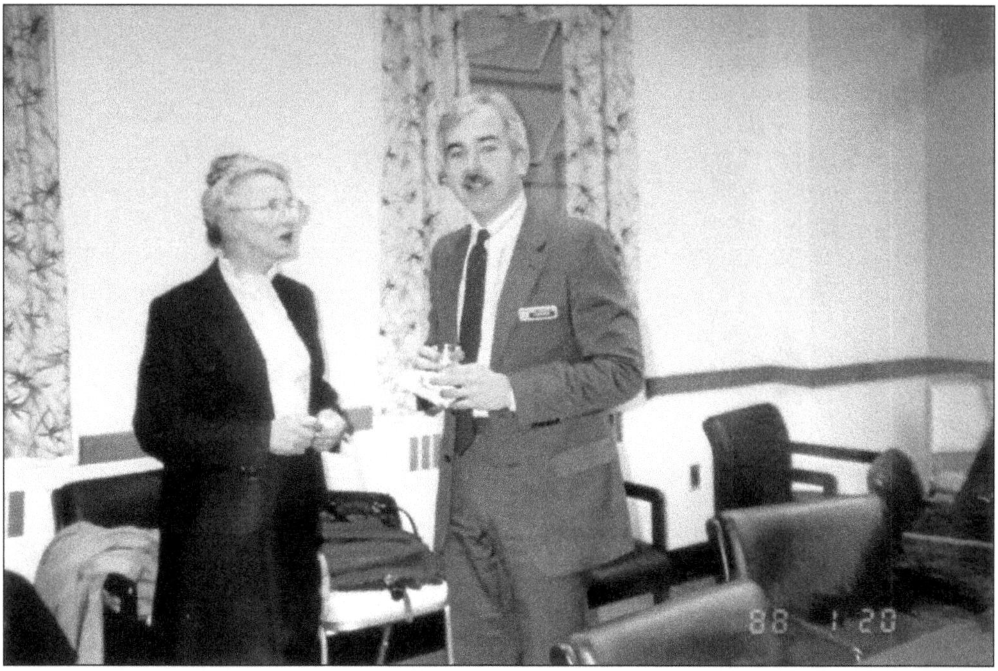

Ann MacDonald retired in 1988 after over 40 years of service. She is seen here with former superintendent Garrell Mullaney at her retirement party in the Kettle Building. Mullaney was the last active superintendent of Norwich Hospital. His successor, Andrew S. Phillips, was brought in primarily to oversee the closing of the hospital. (Courtesy of Ann MacDonald.)

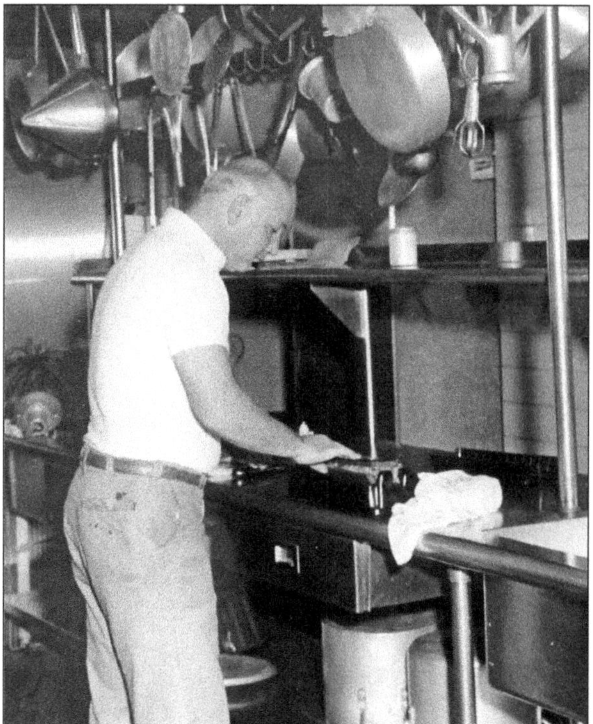

Nick DePolito is another notable and long-running Norwich Hospital retiree. He began his career at Norwich Hospital in 1947. By the end of his career, he was a head cook in the Kettle Building. DePolito stayed with NH for a few more years as a part-time retiree. (Courtesy of Kristen Polci-Parsons.)

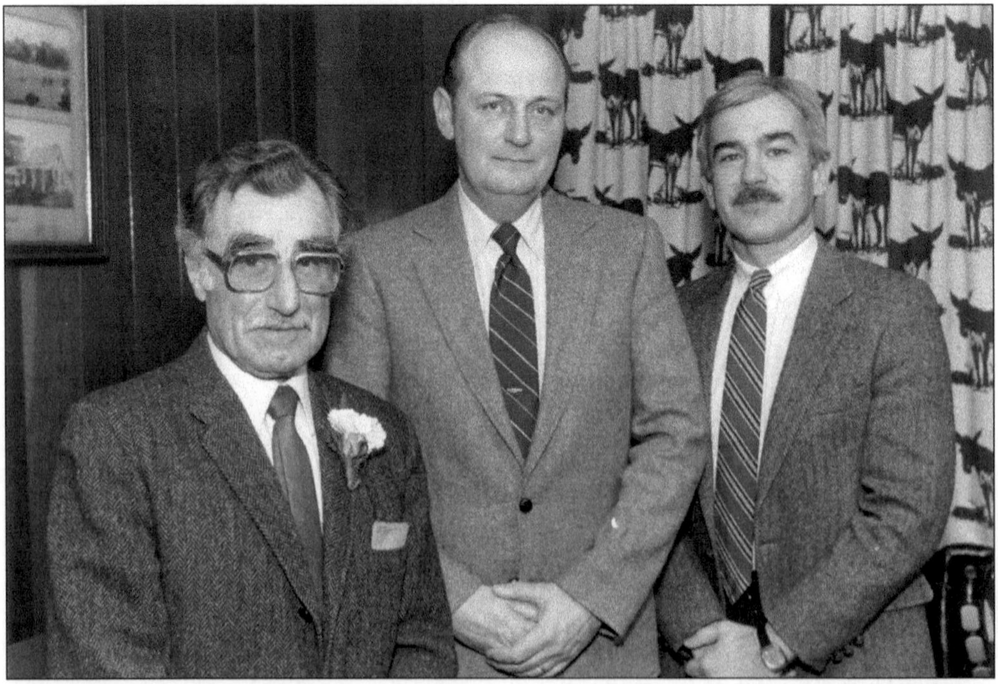

James "Jimmy" John was another of Norwich Hospital's longest running employees and perhaps the most remembered. Jimmy, above on the left, stands with Paul Jette (center) and former NH superintendent Garrell Mullaney during his retirement party in 1987. Jimmy began his career at Norwich Hospital in 1946. During World War II, he suffered from recurring bleeding ulcers that excluded him from military duty. Not wanting to be known as a draft dodger, he took a position in the maintenance department with the intention of staying at the state hospital for a day or two. That turned into a love for his work and Norwich Hospital, where he continued to work on a part-time basis after his retirement. Jimmy was most loved and remembered for always wearing a suit and tie every day. Hundreds of employees fondly remember Jimmy John digging ditches and riding his tractor across the hospital property, proudly wearing his suit and tie. (Courtesy of Jacki John.)

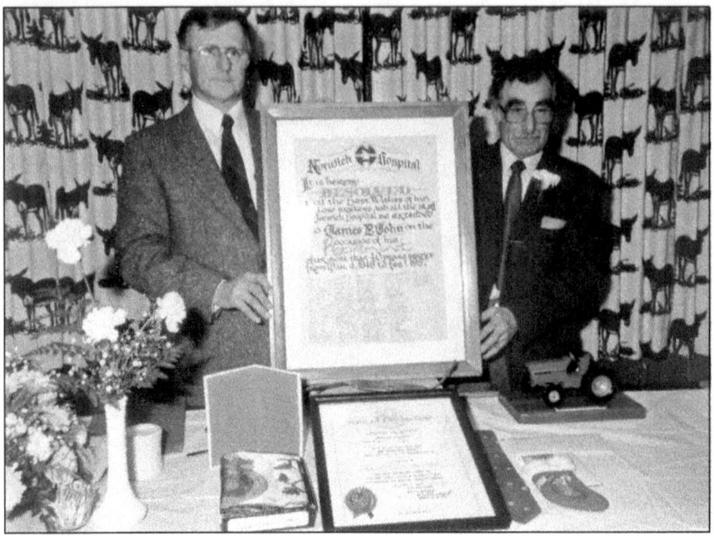

Jimmy John is seen here at his retirement party with Jim Besade (left), an educational instructor at Norwich Hospital. Jimmy was presented with this certificate celebrating his service of over 40 years. (Courtesy of Jacki John.)

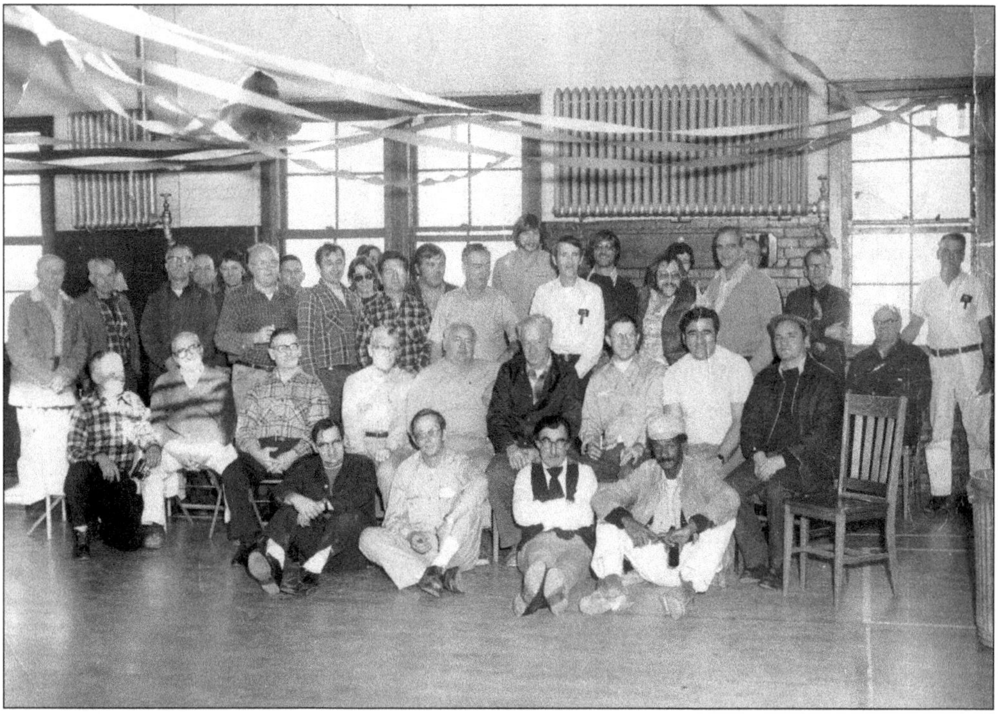

This photograph of Norwich Hospital's maintenance crew was taken during the 1970s. These workers kept Norwich Hospital's grounds immaculate and kept everything running smoothly. Jimmy John is seated on the floor in the first row, second from right. (Courtesy of Jacki John.)

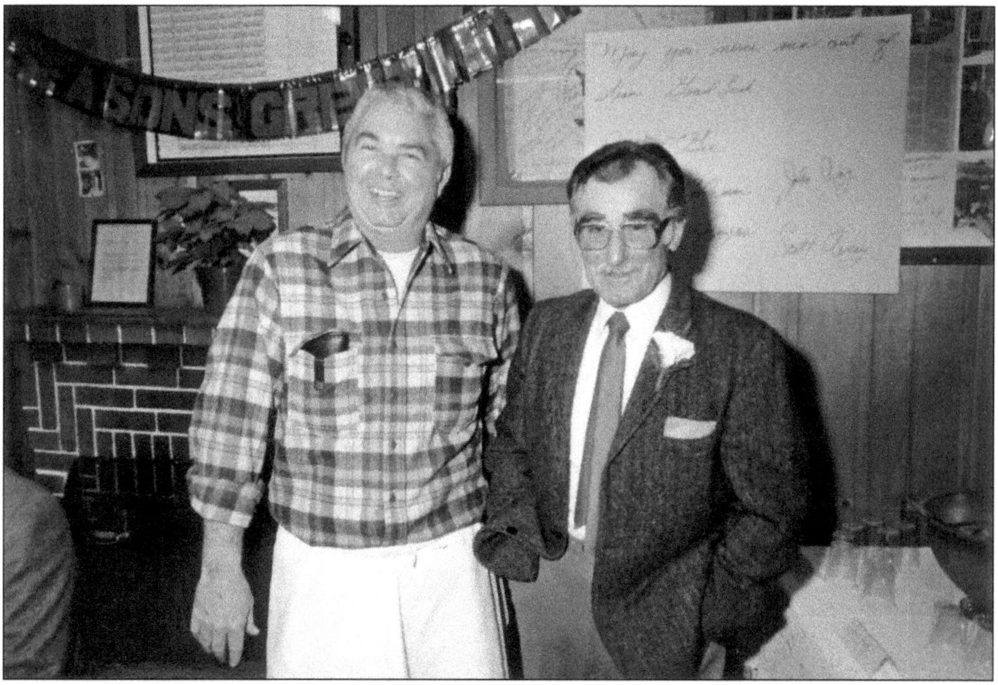

During his retirement party, Jimmy stands beside the head of the Norwich Hospital maintenance department, John Avery. (Courtesy of Jacki John.)

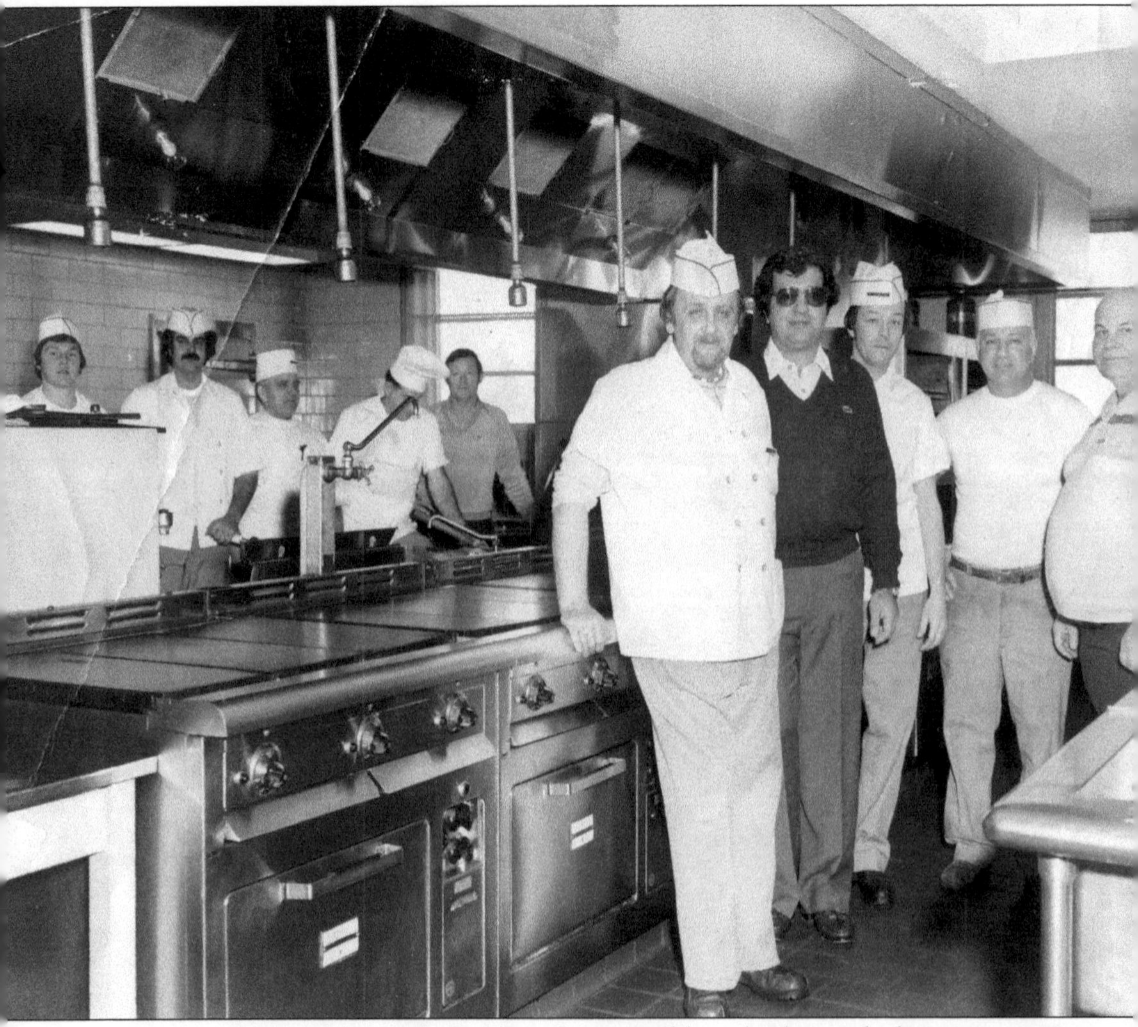

With the opening of the Kettle Building, the original large kitchen and adjoining congregate dining room were closed. All meals for the wards were now prepared in the spacious kitchens inside both the Kettle and Lodge Buildings. Kettle's kitchen staff is pictured here in the late 1970s. From left to right are (first row) Art Sienkowski, Vinny Iacoi, Ralph Johnston, Nick DePolito, and Herman Mainville; (second row) Walter Garnder, Harry Vierra, two unidentified, and Gerry McKeon. (Courtesy of Steve DePolito.)

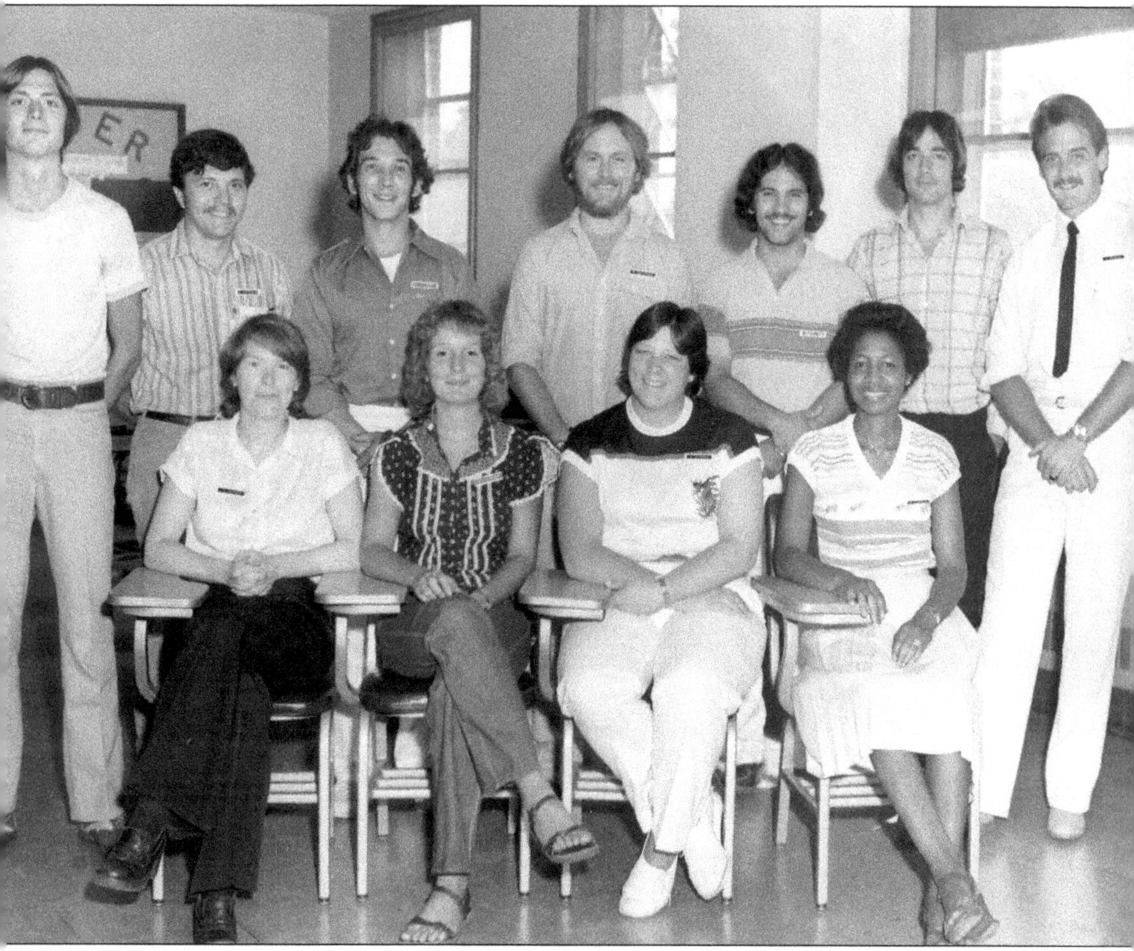

Nick DePolito's son Steve began his mental health career at Norwich Hospital in 1981 as a mental health worker. He is pictured in the back row, third from right. Norwich Hospital had an intensive Nursing Education department for the new psychiatric aides. Around 1985, psychiatric aides were reclassified as mental health workers. Steve DePolito originally worked in the Kettle Building, but later became part of what was called the "float pool" and would eventually have the opportunity to work on every unit at Norwich Hospital. During his career, he learned a great deal of NH's history and became a self-made Norwich Hospital historian. After the hospital closed, he released a video documentary titled *Brewster's Neck: Memories of Norwich State Hospital* to coincide with the 10th anniversary of the hospital's closure. Jimmy John was one of many former employees featured in the video documentary. (Courtesy of Steve DePolito.)

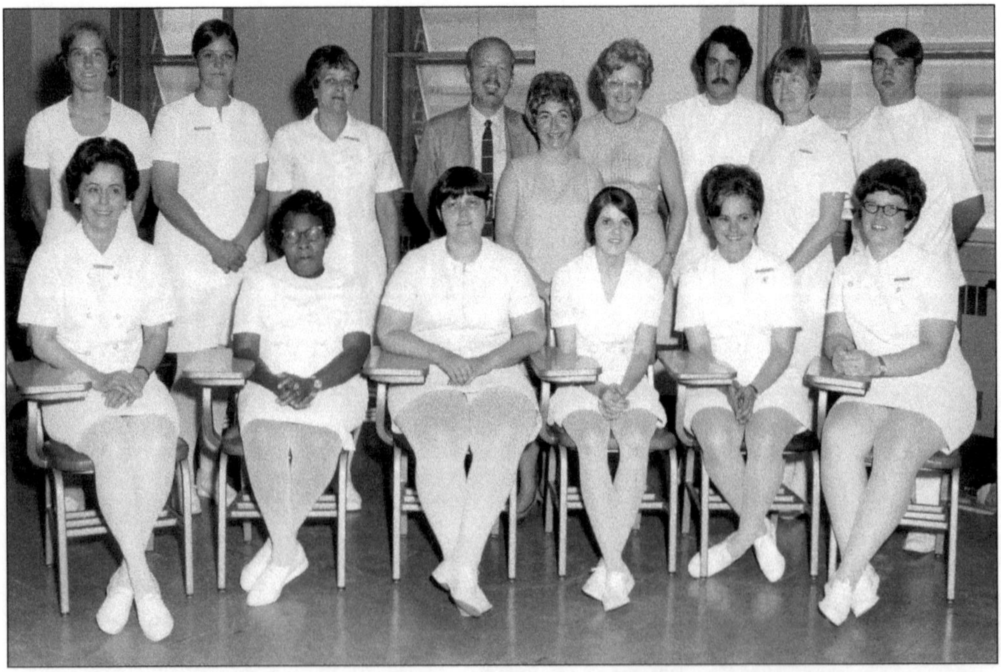

Norwich Hospital's mental health worker courses graduated hundreds of trainees each year. Not everyone who took the courses graduated or continued at Norwich Hospital. Some graduated and took work in different hospitals. Others felt the job was too dangerous. The work environment at Norwich Hospital was ever-changing and often hostile. Workers never knew what they would be walking into at the start of each day. Patients were often agitated, and workers were often injured. Incidents such as patients setting their beds on fire, as seen below, were not uncommon. It was this type of instability that gave birth to the family-like bonds between employees. In the photograph above are, from left to right, (first row) Sabrina Pekawski, Dollie Davis, Audrey Zaratkiewicz, Jean Gonzales, Penny Walters, and Linda Smith; (second row) Karen Hantsche, Patricia Clifford, Alice Joelson, Supt. Dr. Morgan Martin, Beverely Greenwood, Dorothy Douglas (director of nursing education), James Riden, Rejeanne Thornton, and Allyn Fontaine. (Above, courtesy of Steve DePolito; below, courtesy of Kristen Polci-Parsons.)

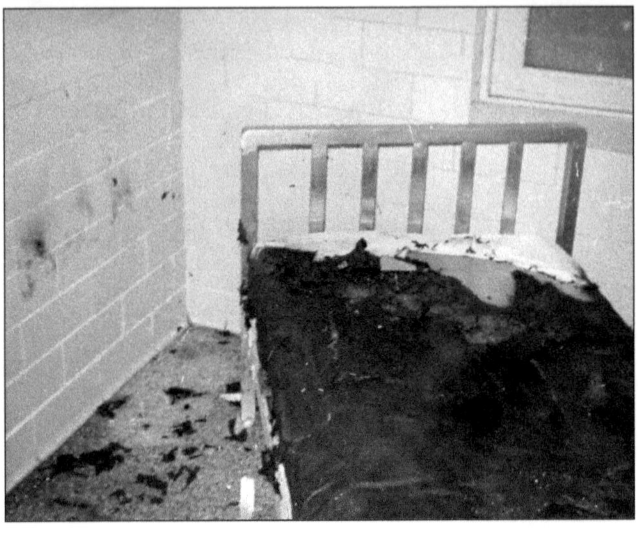

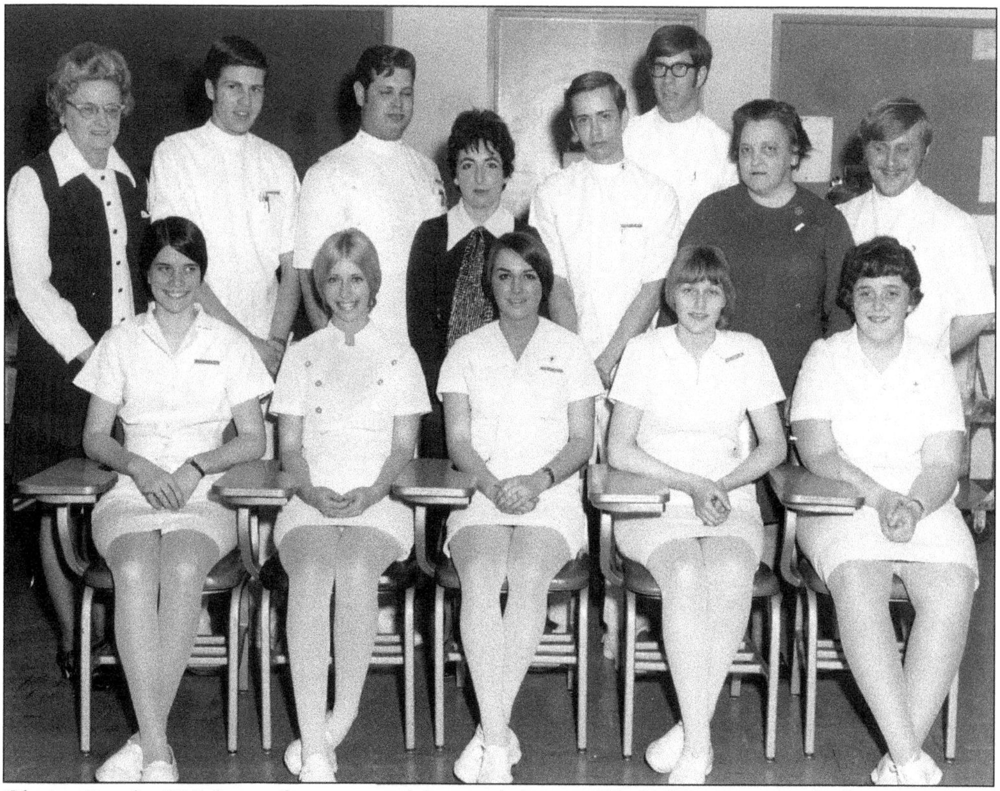

Clarice Proulx, RN, (second row, second from right) was a World War II nurse who began working at Norwich Hospital in the 1950s. By the mid-1960s, she was an instructor in the nursing education department. She educated students in psychiatric nursing care for 20 years. Proulx was a beloved instructor and was remembered fondly by many. This photograph shows one of her graduating classes from 1970. From left to right are (first row) Martha Coulombe, Sandra Ross, Renee Lozon, Carol Fontaine, and Diane Pawlik; (second row) Dorothy Douglas (director of nursing education), Kenneth Gibson, Anthony Williams, Beverly Greenwood (instructor), Kenneth Parizo, William Cawthra, Proulx, and Joseph Bielawkski. (Courtesy of Steve DePolito.)

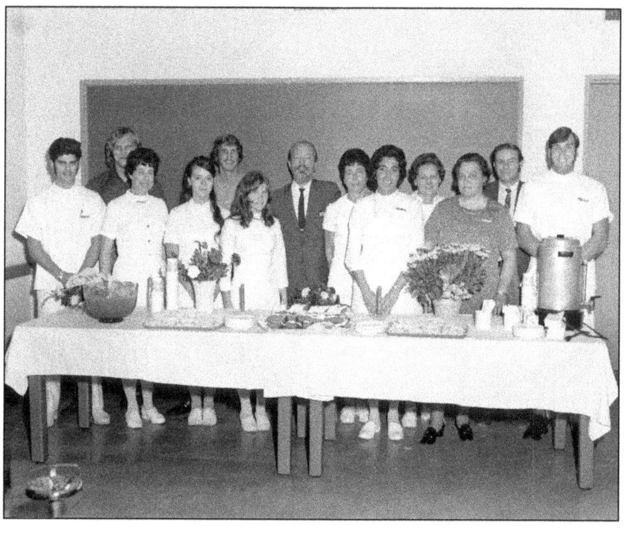

Proulx's Psychiatric Aide Training Group No. 28, from 1970, is shown here in a classroom in the Kettle Building. Proulx is second from right, and Supt. Dr. Morgan Martin is seventh from right. (Courtesy of Steve DePolito.)

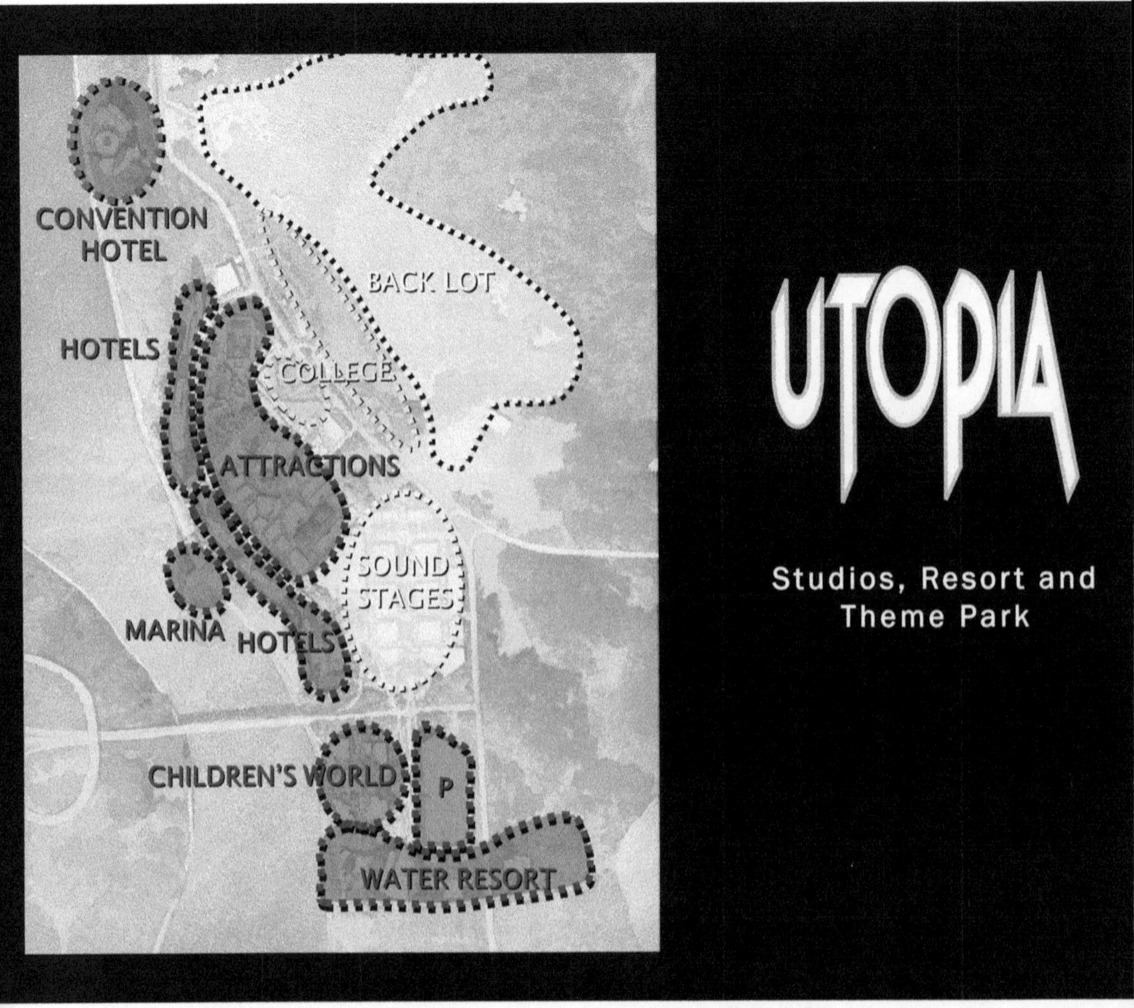

Following the closure of Norwich Hospital, redevelopment ideas and proposals began to pour in. Located across the Thames River from the newly opened Mohegan Sun Casino in 1996 and just a few miles from Foxwoods Resort and Casino, numerous companies wanted to take advantage of this prime real estate. Three Rivers College proposed moving some of its campus to two buildings on the Norwich Hospital property, but that did not come to fruition. In 2003, developer Utopia Studios expressed heavy interest in redeveloping the old hospital property into a fantastic large-scale family-oriented theme park complete with hotels and a marina. Utopia also boasted promises of the site being home to movie and television studios. This 2005 image depicts Utopia's proposed master plan for reuse of the Norwich Hospital property. Utopia wanted to renovate and incorporate many of the old hospital buildings for an onsite college, hotel, and central attractions. After several years of negotiations, the deal was ultimately rejected by the State of Connecticut because Utopia failed to deliver proper documentation of its plans. (Author's collection.)

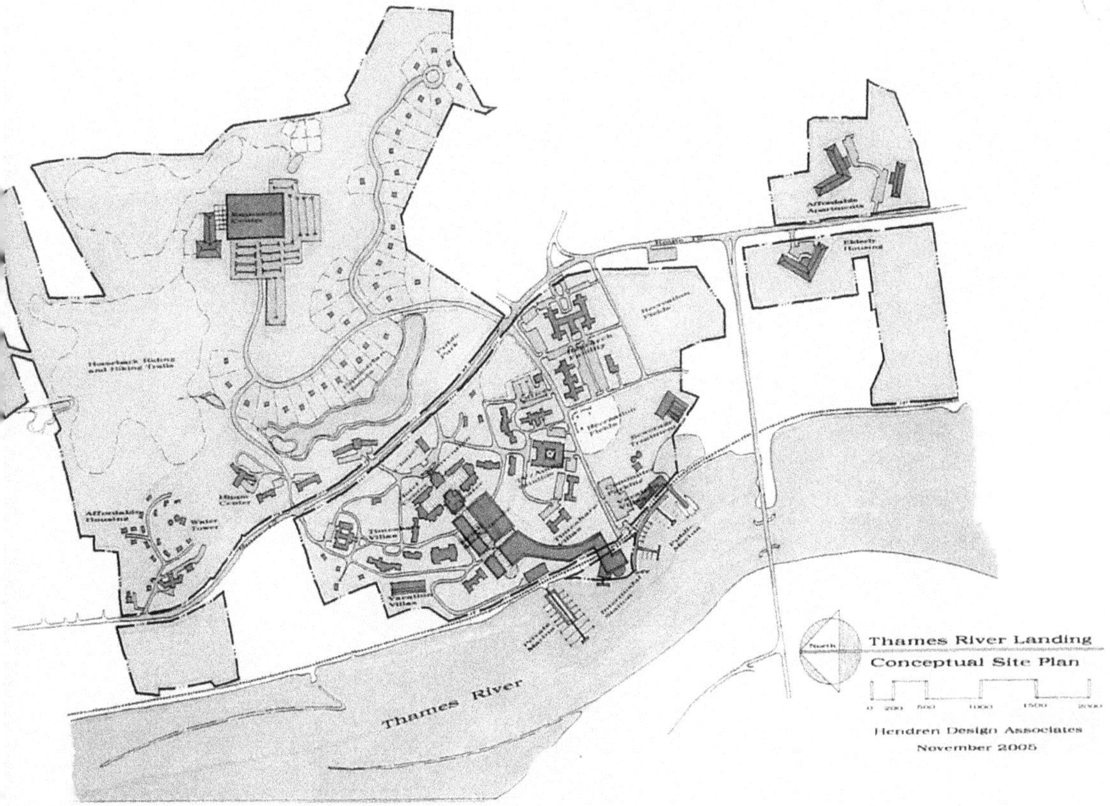

Thames River Landing was another hospital property redevelopment proposal that landed on the table in 2005. Thames River Landing Corp idealized the renovation and reuse of a majority of the hospital buildings for an equestrian center, hotel and convention center, marketplace with hotel accommodations, and elderly housing. It envisioned using the Administration Building as a grand entrance to a unique hotel facility comprised of the Salmon, Awl, Bell, Brigham, Woodward, and Stedman Buildings. Thames River Landing deemed the grand theater a "diamond in the rough," and wanted to polish that diamond and restore it to near its original beauty. But like Utopia, this deal never saw the light of day. After these failed attempts, the hospital sat in limbo for the next four years. In 2009, the town of Preston bought 400 acres of the property from the state for $1. The town promised that it would do what the state failed to do for 13 years: demolish the buildings they felt were an eyesore to the area and successfully redevelop the Norwich State Hospital property. (Author's collection.)

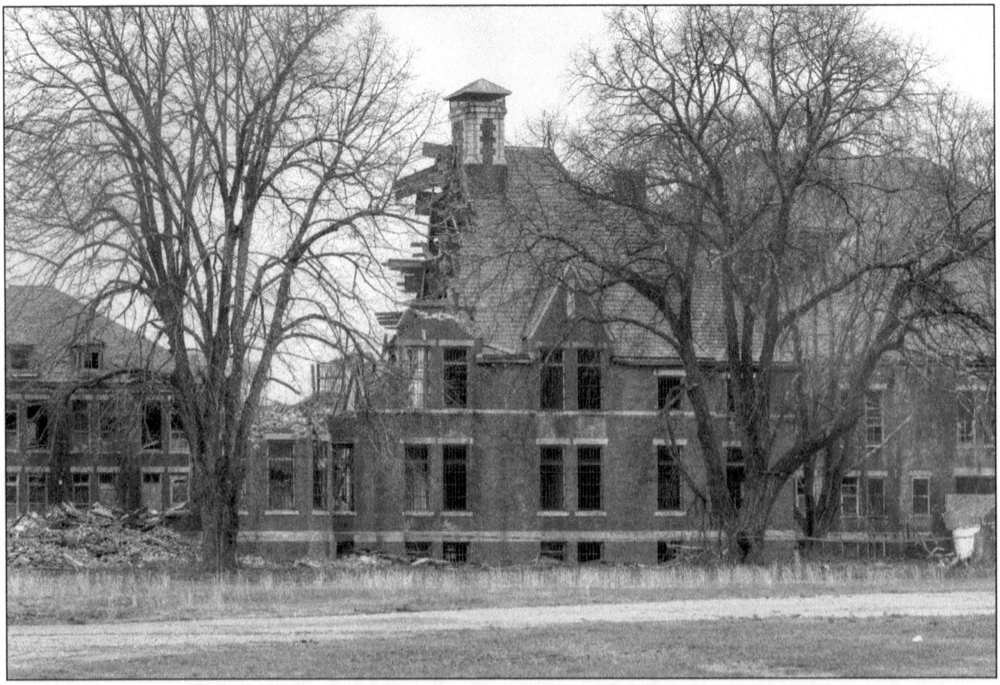

After years of failure to initiate redevelopment of the Norwich State Hospital property, demolition of the hospital buildings again began to make headlines in 2010 as the town of Preston solidified its promise to move forward. Numerous applications for grants to fund demolition of the hospital buildings took three years to be approved. In December 2011, demolition began at the rear of the property with the powerhouse and laundry buildings. Demolition moved roadside and became the local hot topic with the destruction of the first and oldest ward buildings on the campus: Salmon and Awl. Wooden planks stick out from the partially demolished Salmon Building, pictured here in March 2012. Salmon was demolished in a little over a week, with Awl and the chapel immediately after. (Author's collection.)

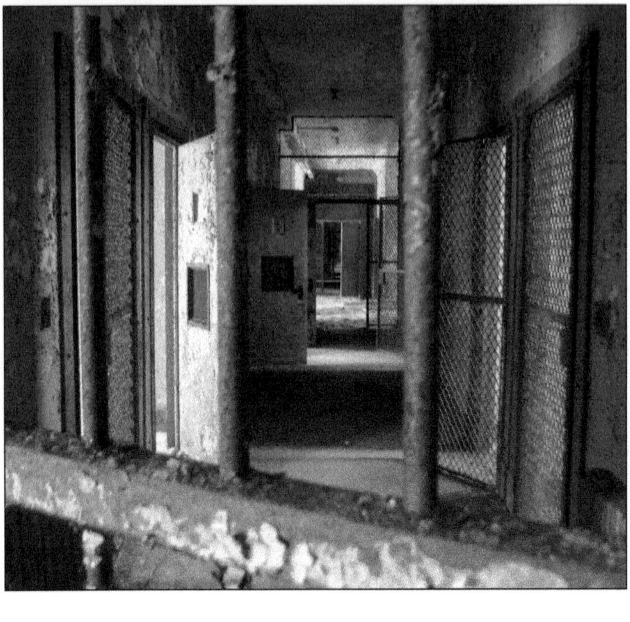

The cold iron bars and caged doors on the cells of Salmon II were fodder for decades of local myths of patient abuses and wild horror stories that gained Norwich State Hospital unfitting infamy, further tarnishing the public's view of psychiatric hospitals. The demolition of this famous hallway buried the era of mistreatment that had always been a hindrance to NSH: Patients only being afforded accommodations like this at the hands of legislative misappropriations rather than receiving the benefit of facilities constructed specifically for their care. (Author's collection.)

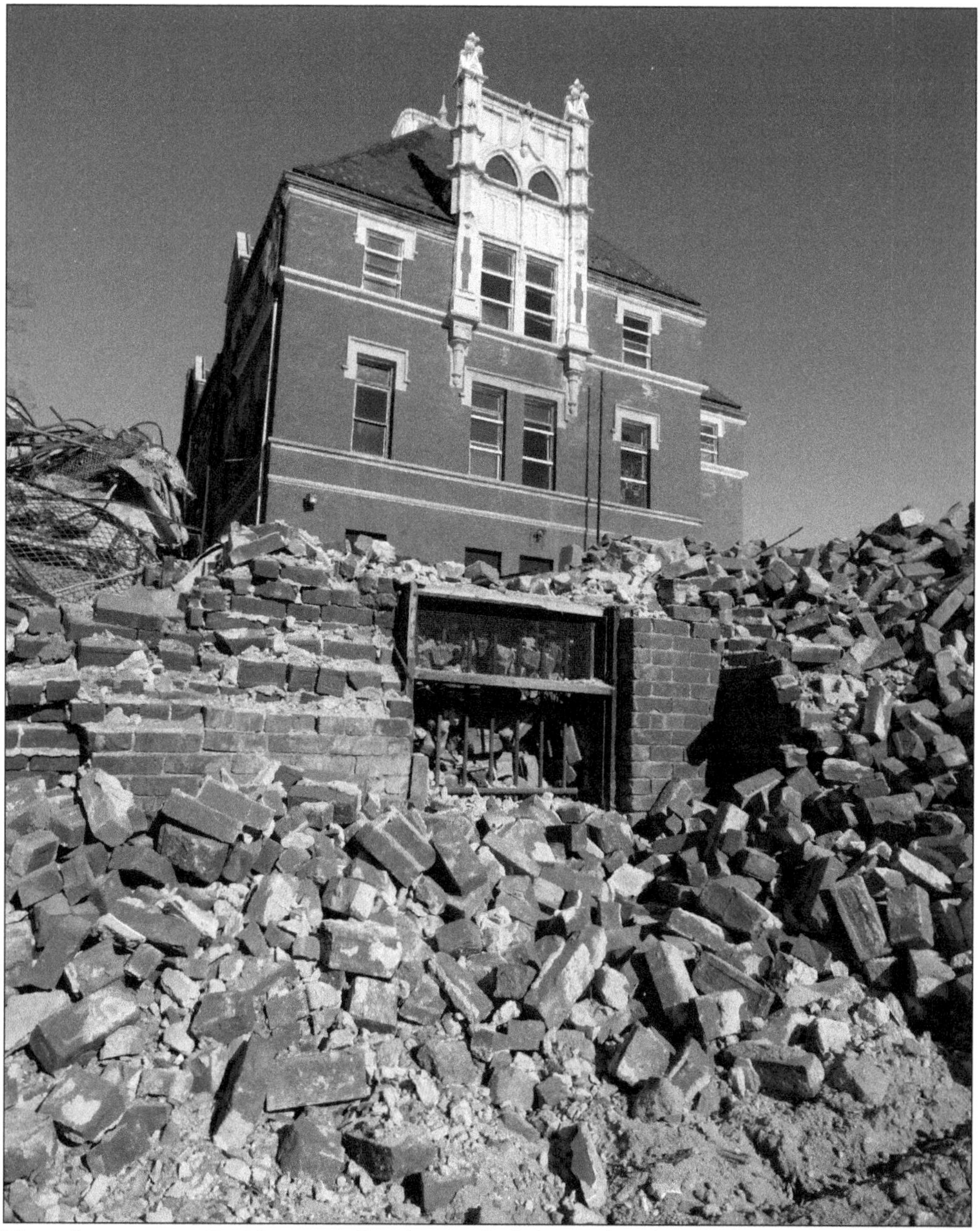

The Administration Building sits tall and unscathed above a lone basement window of the Salmon Building with its iron bars still intact. Salmon's 108-year old broken bricks crumbled down into what was its basement. As demolition moved forward in 2012, the sight of building after building falling at the hands of the wrecking ball became too heartbreaking for former employees to bear. Many stopped driving down Route 12 altogether to avoid the emotional trauma. Once the public learned the Administration Building was to be spared, former employees and the public expressed high interest in what the future held for the building. Since the onset of demolition, concrete preservation plans for the Administration Building have been left up in the air, and hopes for the building to be used to honor and recognize thousands spanning nearly 100 years of service remain in the balance. (Author's collection.)

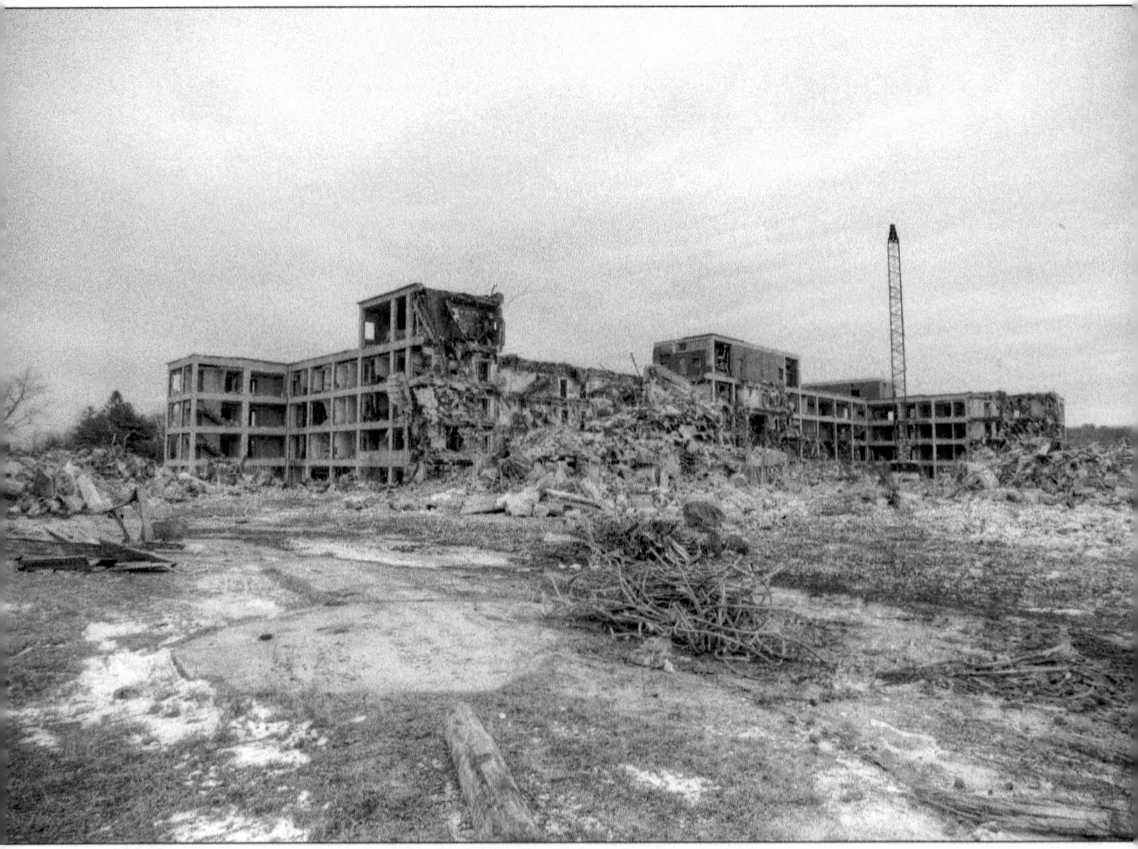

One by one, buildings on the Norwich State Hospital campus were reduced to piles of twisted metal and broken bricks. It was a painful sight for former employees and their families to see, passing down Route 12 as demolition slowly moved forward over a period of six years. The Kettle Building, pictured during demolition in 2015, is now nothing more than an empty field. The staff-planted daffodils, which signified the start of every spring season, no longer rise from the ground in front of where the building stood. To some, the sight of the empty hospital property is one of joy and anticipated rebirth. To others, the plain, flat land will always hold the memories of their lives, careers, family, and friends lived out in the buildings they called home. (Author's collection.)

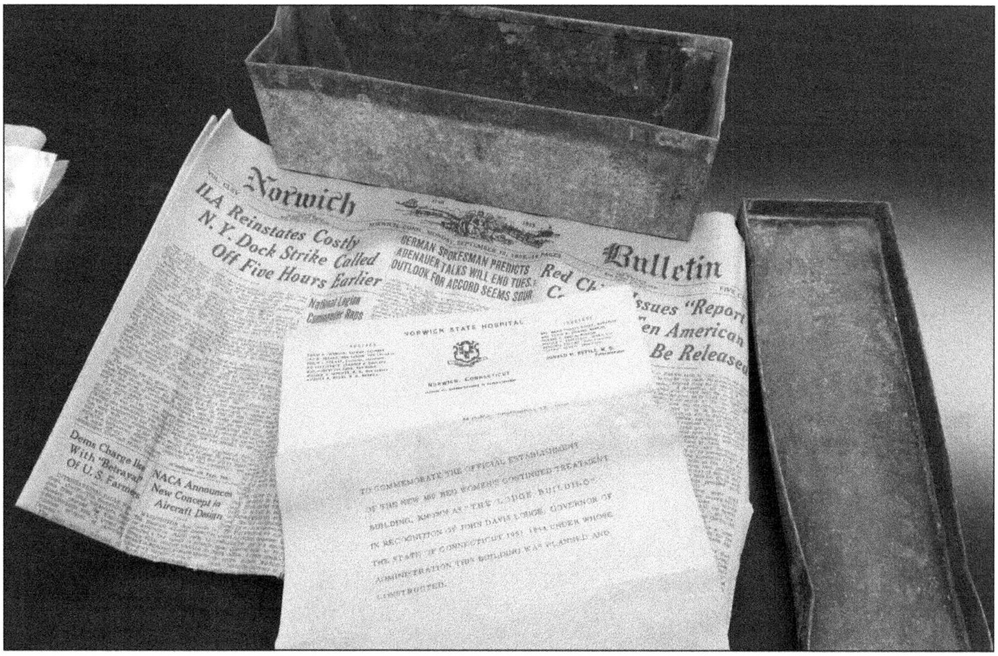
Norwich Bulletin
ILA Reinstates Costly
N.Y. Dock Strike Called
Off Five Hours Earlier
German Spokesman Predicts
Adenauer Talks Will End Tues.;
Outlook for Accord Seems Sour
NACA Announces
New Concept in
Aircraft Design
Norwich State Hospital
Norwich, Connecticut

During the demolition of the Lodge Building in 2014, a metal box containing documents was discovered. This time capsule, now dented and rusted, had been buried within the walls of the building. A letter commemorating the official establishment of the Lodge Building (shown in full on the next page), a copy of the *Norwich Bulletin* dated September 12, 1955, and a hand-written letter in blue ink, which was deteriorated beyond legibility, were among the box's contents. (Author's collection.)

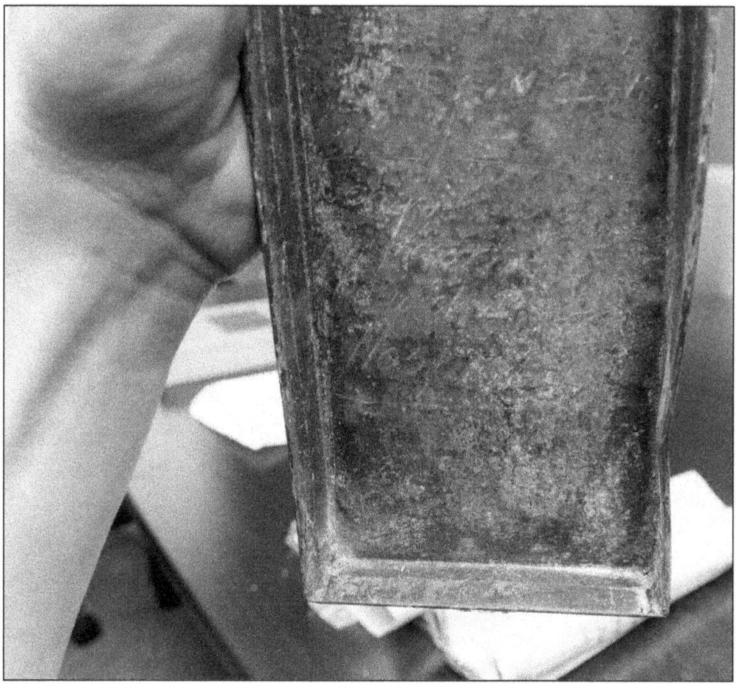

Close examination of the time capsule box revealed that it was constructed in the hospital's metals shop and was inscribed by all those contributing to its contents and placement within the building. Due to deterioration, the inscriptions are almost impossible to read, but the words, "Norwich State Hospital," can be made out. (Author's collection.)

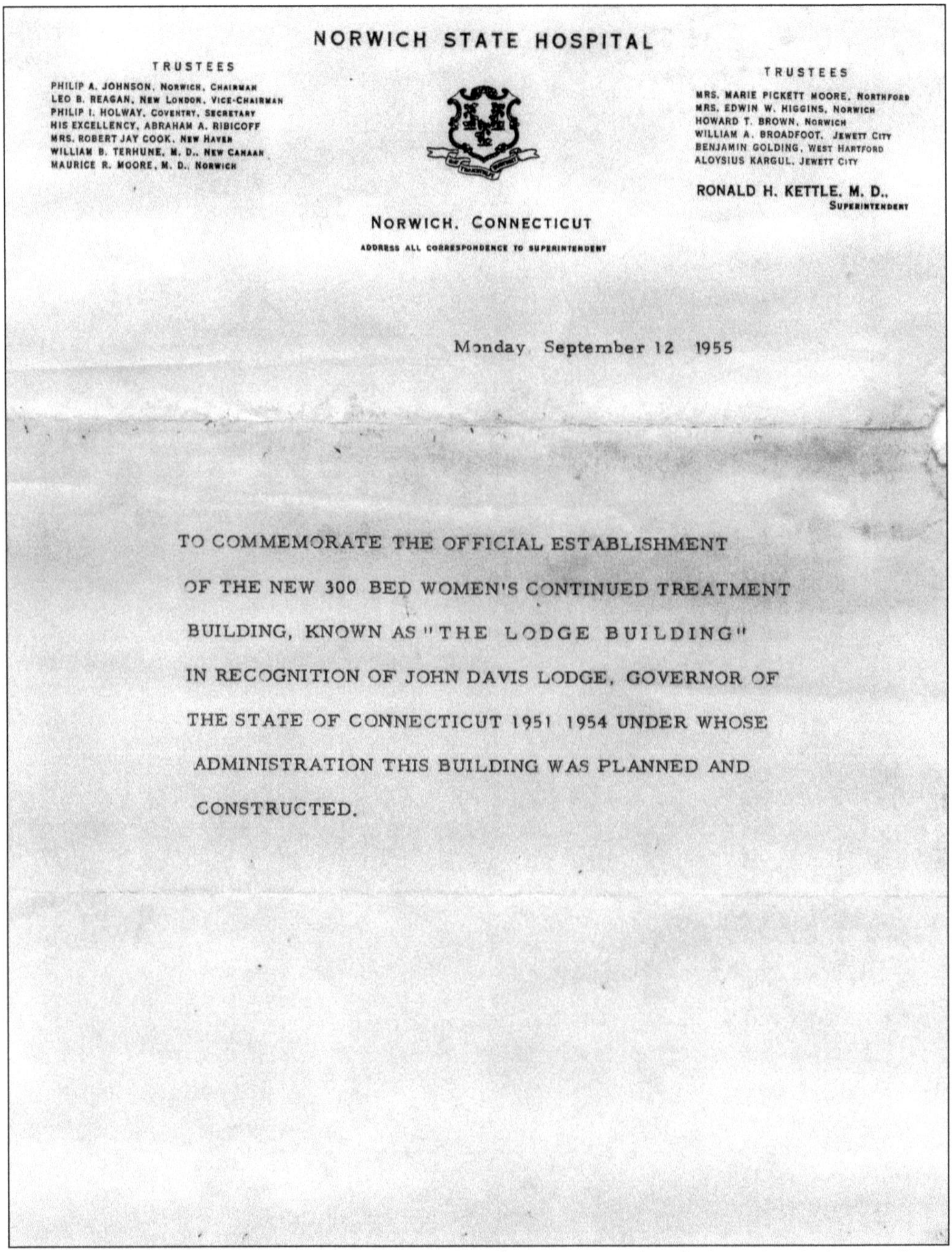

NORWICH STATE HOSPITAL

RONALD H. KETTLE, M. D.,
SUPERINTENDENT

NORWICH, CONNECTICUT

ADDRESS ALL CORRESPONDENCE TO SUPERINTENDENT

Monday September 12 1955

TO COMMEMORATE THE OFFICIAL ESTABLISHMENT
OF THE NEW 300 BED WOMEN'S CONTINUED TREATMENT
BUILDING, KNOWN AS "THE LODGE BUILDING"
IN RECOGNITION OF JOHN DAVIS LODGE, GOVERNOR OF
THE STATE OF CONNECTICUT 1951 1954 UNDER WHOSE
ADMINISTRATION THIS BUILDING WAS PLANNED AND
CONSTRUCTED.

Bearing the same date as the copy of the *Norwich Bulletin* discovered in the box, this dedication letter commemorates the official establishment of the John Lodge Building. The time capsule was buried within the walls of the Lodge Building on Monday, September 12, 1955. (Author's collection.)

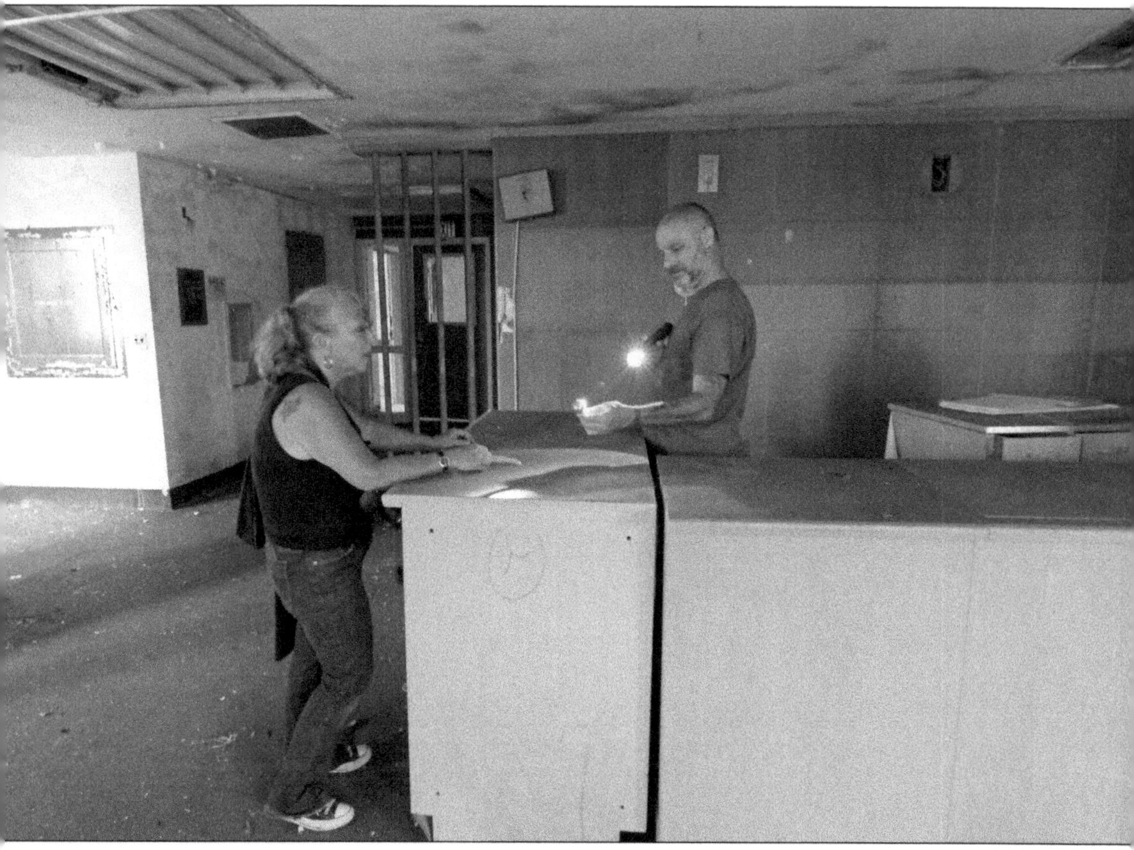

Fifteen years after closure, a venture back into the buildings they spent so many years of their lives working in was like uncovering a time capsule in itself for former workers Patty Nichols and Steven Falade. Nichols (left) was a social worker in the Kettle Building and left Norwich Hospital in 1995 before it closed. Falade (right) was a subcontractor who serviced Norwich Hospital's telephone systems. Falade had always been intrigued by Nichols each time he heard her name paged over the hospital's PA system. Falade had never seen Nichols, but had to know who she was because she was paged so frequently. When he finally saw her skipping down the hall of the Russell Building, where his work was based out of, it was love at first sight. They were married a year later. Their journey back inside the buildings where they met and worked was a surrealist's dream. They are pictured in the Kettle library, just down the hall from Nichols's office, examining small remnants left behind. (Author's collection.)

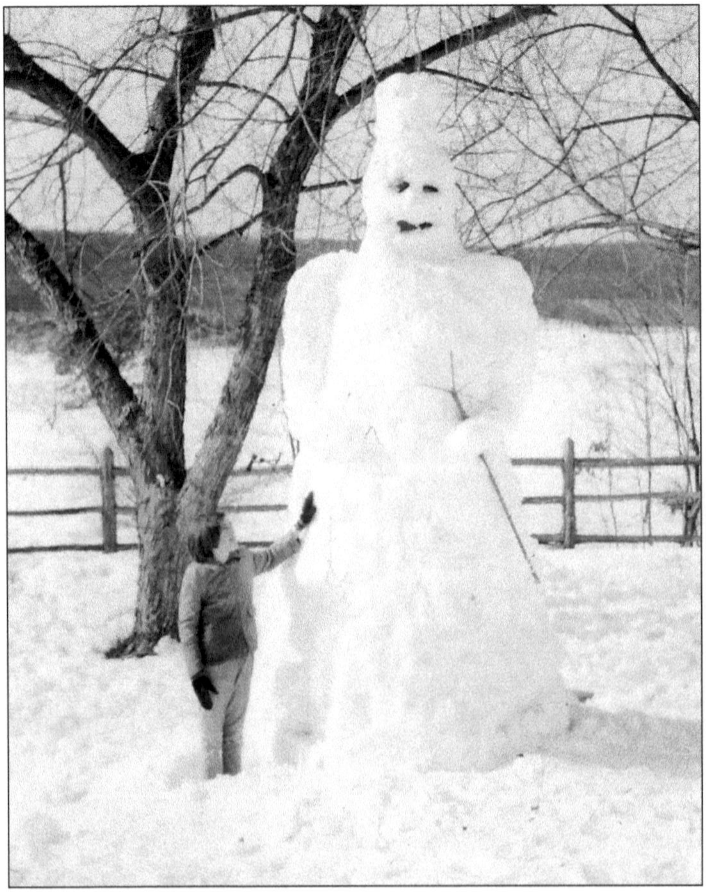

Adults were not the only people whose lives were engulfed in the state hospital lifestyle. Hundreds of children were inducted into state hospital life from birth or from the "normal" world. The Lippitt Building was the site of numerous births of children to both staff and patients. Dorothy Burns, pictured at left at age 11 in 1961 with her snowman Igor, was one of six children of assistant superintendent Warren Burns. The Burns family lived on campus in Cottage No. 2, behind the Lippitt Building (shown below in 1961). (Both, courtesy of Allan Burns.)

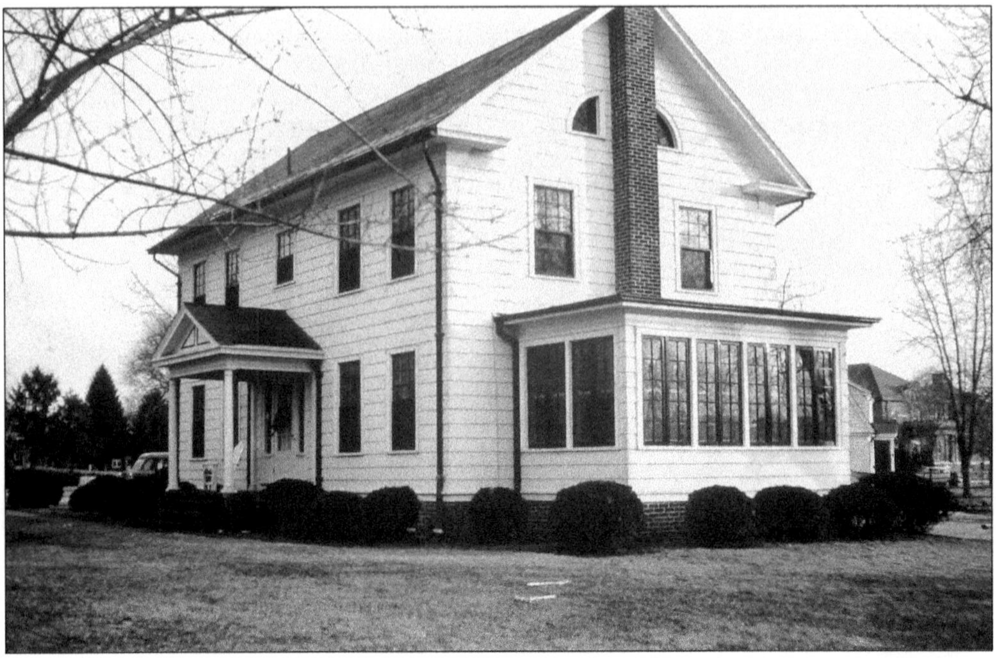

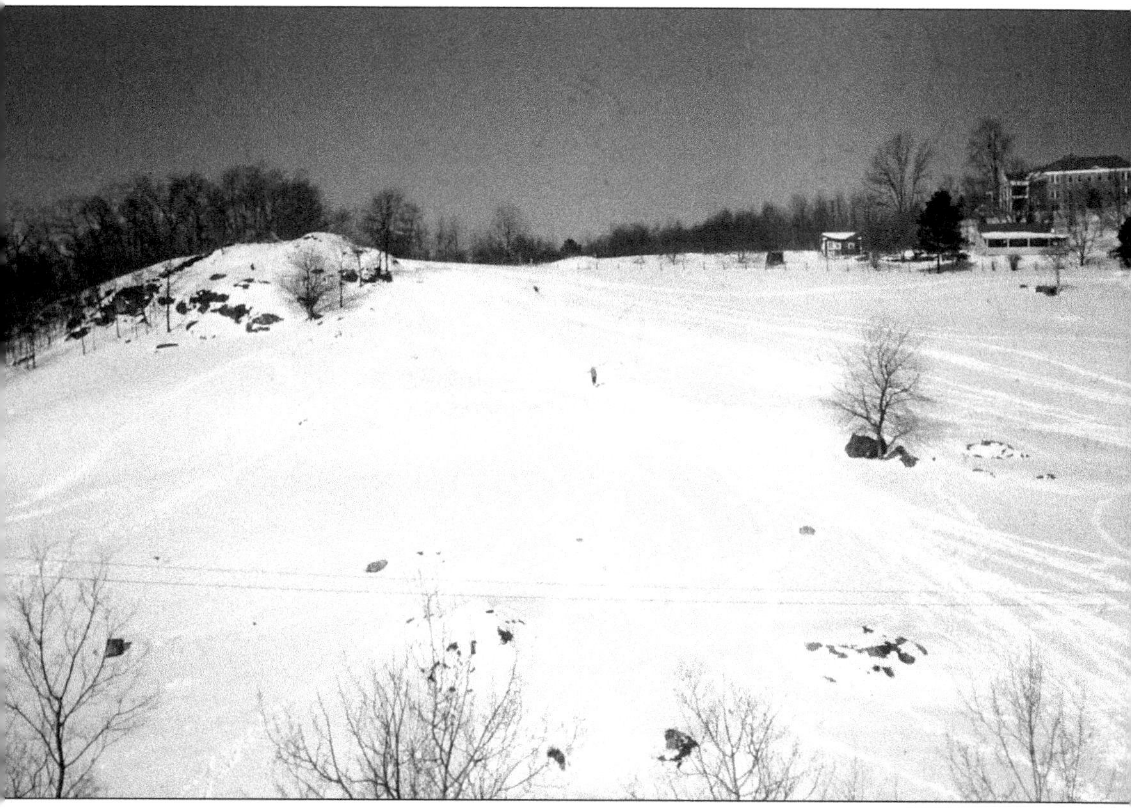

Growing up at the state hospital was different from growing up elsewhere. The stigmatism against mental illness affected children who grew up on state hospital grounds negatively. Parents were hesitant and often refused to allow their children to visit friends who lived at state hospitals due to irrational fears of "the crazies." Dorothy Burns's sister Carol remembers swimming as a child at the state hospital pond with her childhood friends who were scared by patients also swimming in the pond that day. Carol remembers other times patients affected her childhood, as she recalls in her poem about youth on the grounds of Norwich State Hospital: "I met patients on the mend, who came to clean our house / One who was followed by tricksters; / One who gave my practiced mother / A run for her money at crosswords and cryptograms. / I loved her. She was sweet and kind. / She locked me in the bathroom with her to protect me, / Unable to articulate how she knew I was being harmed." Otherwise, fun winter days skiing down Wheeler Hill across the street from the Bryan Building, like in this photograph from 1961, were the norm, as for everyone else. (Courtesy of Allan Burns.)

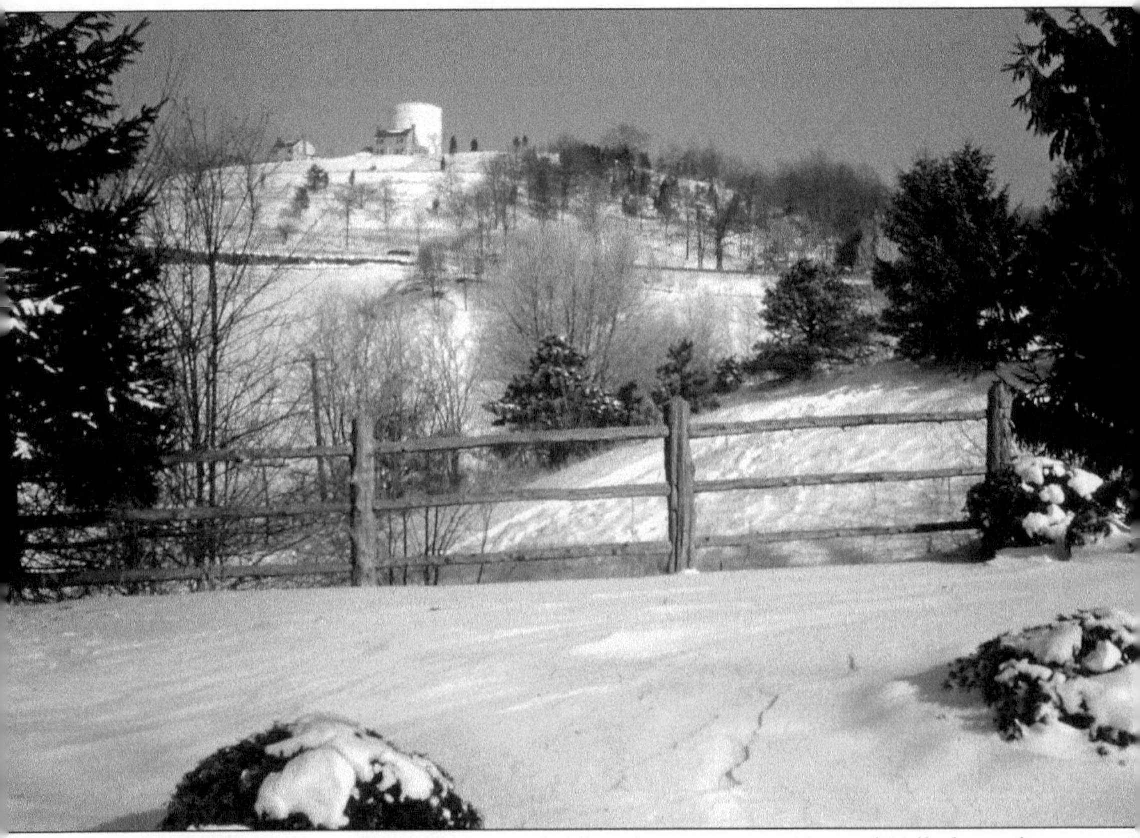

Carol McDermott reminisced about her childhood memories on Hospital Hill, shown here in 1961: "The road, which still climbs up to "the hill," / Where a small community half-circles a water tower; / A water tower I once climbed on a dare / To stand on the edge looking down on our kingdom. / The sloping hills where we picked berries / To eat and box and sell to our neighbors. / We were wild and juicy like the blackberries. / Our fingers stained and pricked, making our bucks. / On the other side of our house, / Separated by trees and closer to the world of normal / Stood the house of the then-Superintendent, Dr. Kettle. / Mrs. Kettle bought two velvet Jesus pictures I purchased / Through a comic book and sold door to door." Her childhood memories are no different from any other child's in any walk of life. (Courtesy of Allan Burns.)

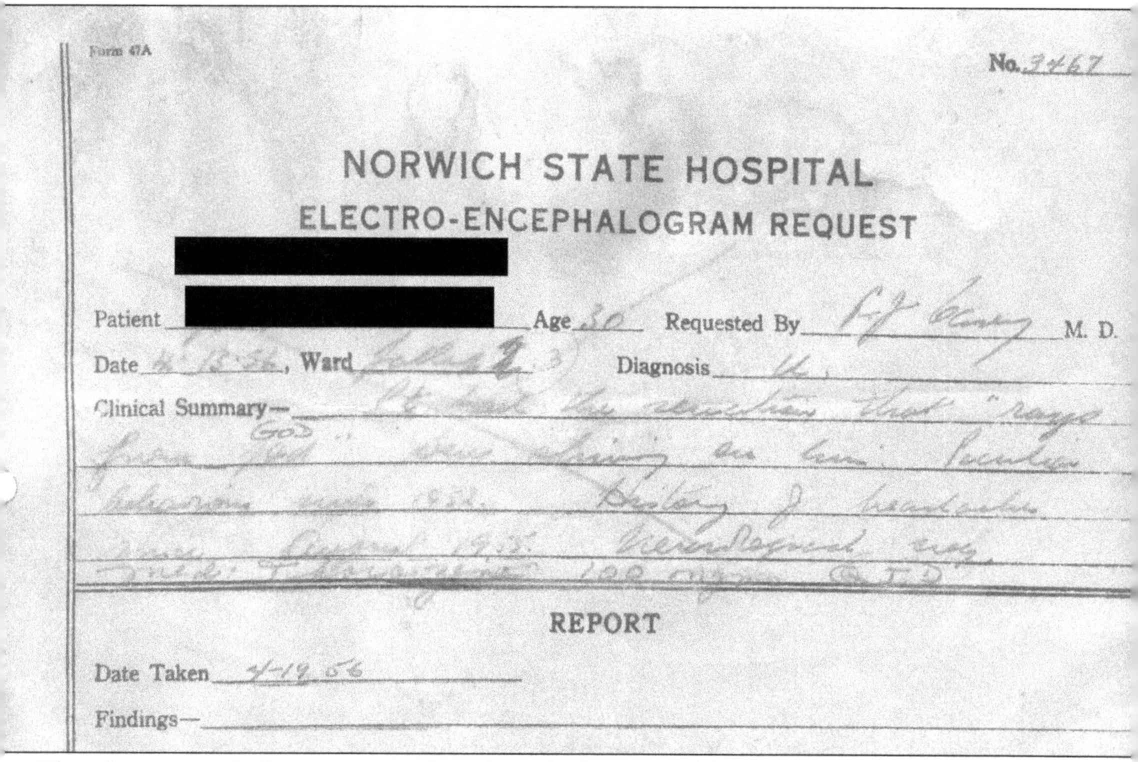

Form 47A

No. 3467

NORWICH STATE HOSPITAL

ELECTRO-ENCEPHALOGRAM REQUEST

Patient ______ Age 30 Requested By ______ M. D.

Date ______, Ward ______ Diagnosis ______

Clinical Summary—

REPORT

Date Taken 4-19-56

Findings—

This electro-encephalogram request form from the Lippitt Building in 1956 reads, "Pt had the revelation that "rays from God" were shining on him. Peculiar behavior since 1952. History of headaches since August 1955. Neurological: reg. Med: Thorazine 100mg QID." Through a child's eyes, patients like this were fodder for curious young minds. Carol McDermott wrote, "Once I snuck into my father's study / To read the notes about a man who thought he was Jesus. / He made an intelligent case. / I asked my dad how did he know this man wasn't Jesus. / I was chastised for snooping. / I thought at that time that the shrinks were weirder / Than their patients." (Author's collection.)

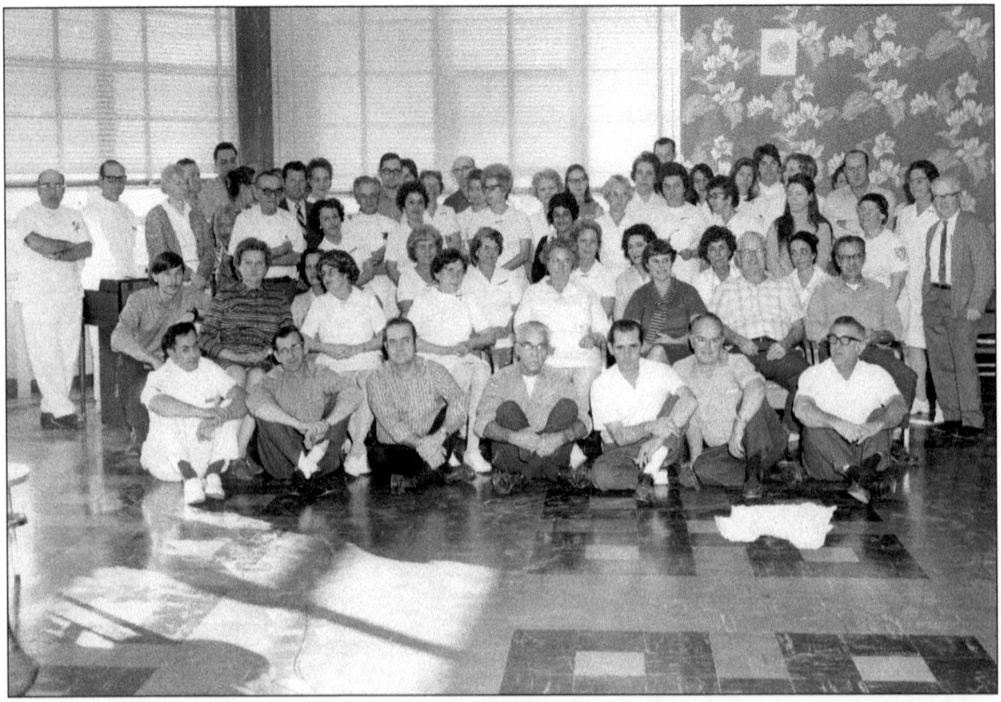

The dedication and hard work from the multitude of generations of selfless souls who graced the grounds and the halls of Norwich Hospital will never be forgotten. From the large groups of mental health workers like those above in the Russell Building Solarium to Captain McGowan and Sergeant Romano of Norwich Hospital law enforcement below around 1960, the tremendous legacy and memories of Norwich Hospital's employees will proudly live on to be told time and again for generations to come. (Above, courtesy of Steve DePolito; below, courtesy of Patti Daniels.)

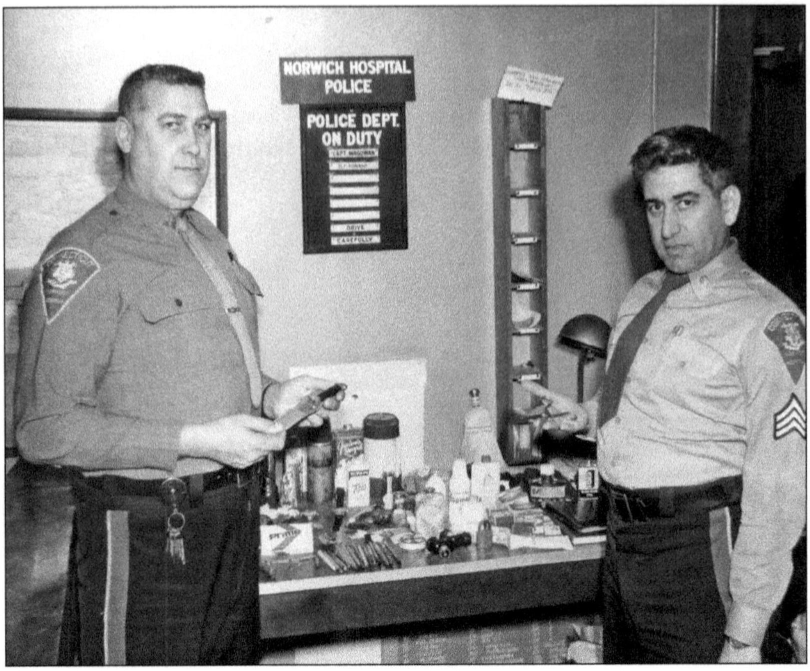

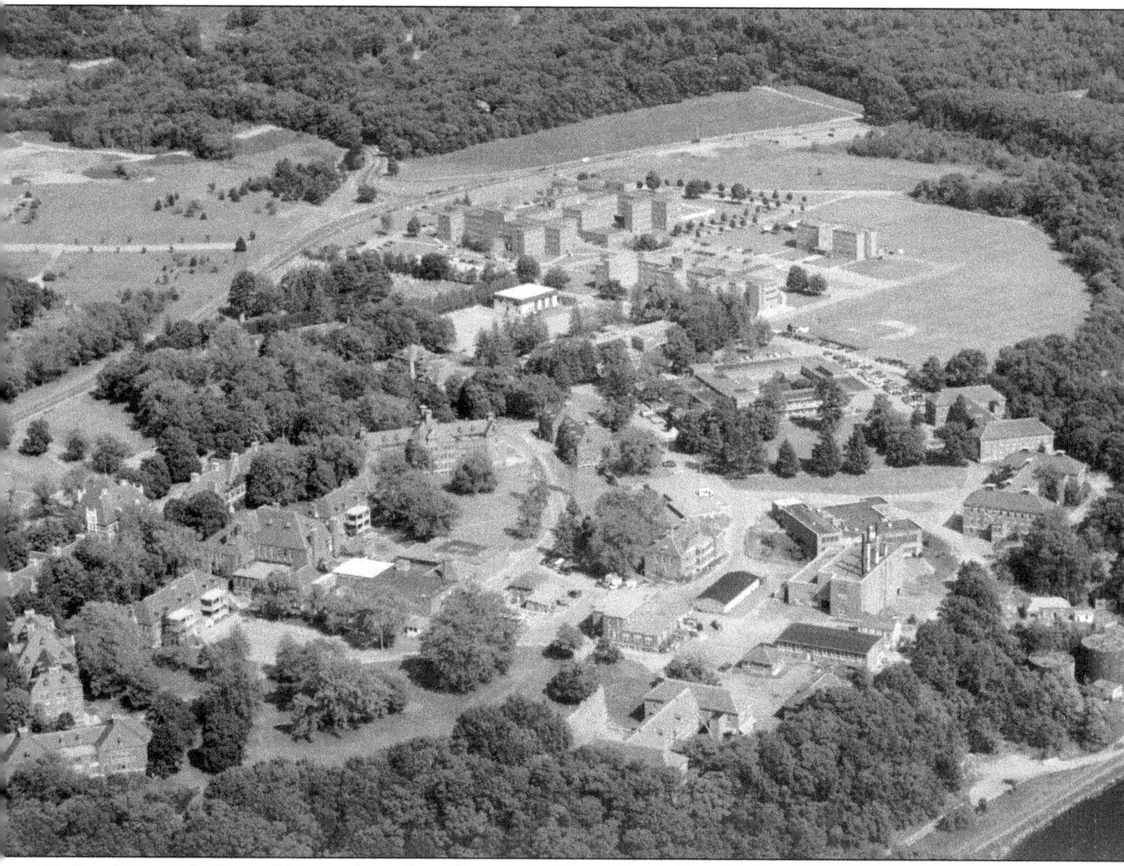

Today, Norwich State Hospital sits largely as an empty plot of land awaiting redevelopment. No matter what the future holds for this area of Preston, Connecticut, known as Brewster's Neck, this land will forever be known and preserved in the memories of many as it appears in this aerial view from the mid-1990s, shortly before the hospital closed—as Norwich State Hospital. Carol McDermott wrote in 2012: "And down the hill is the heart of the hospital— / The renowned and venerable Norwich State. / Licked by the Thames River on one side / Bordered by my beloved woods and pond on the other." (Author's collection.)

www.ingramcontent.com/pod-product-compliance
Lightning Source LLC
LaVergne TN
LVHW070820030926
847199LV00039B/508
* 9 7 8 1 4 6 7 1 2 9 6 2 6 *